MANAGING TYPE · II DIABETES

Your Invitation to a Healthier Lifestyle

Arlene Monk, R.D., C.D.E.

Jan Pearson, B.A.N., R.N., C.D.E.

Priscilla Hollander, M.D., Ph.D.

Richard M. Bergenstal, M.D.

IDC Publishing

Minneapolis

This book cannot serve as a substitute for a physician's medical care. The information it contains cannot be used to diagnose medical conditions or prescribe treatment.

Acknowledgments

The authors wish to thank Barb Barry, M.S., R.D., C.D.E., Joe Nelson, M.A., L.P., and Gloria Wood, Ph.D., L.P. for their assistance in writing this book. A special thank you to the reviewers and all the staff of International Diabetes Center for their support and encouragement.

IDC Publishing
3800 Park Nicollet Boulevard
Minneapolis, Minnesota 55416-2699, U.S.A.
(612) 993-3393

Printed in the United States of America
10   9   8   7   6   5   4   3   2   1

Editor: Karol Carstensen
Copy Editor: Sara Frueh
Production Manager: Gail Devery
Cover and text design: Lois Stanfield, LightSource Images, St. Paul
Illustrations in Chapter 11: Hetty Mitchell

Library of Congress Cataloging-in-Publication Data
Managing type II diabetes: your invitation to a healthier lifestyle/Arlene Monk
. . . [et al.].
    p.   cm.
    Originally published: Wayzata, Minn.: DCI Pub., 1988.
    Includes bibliographical references and index.
    ISBN 1-885115-26-1 (alk. paper)
    1. Non-insulin-dependent diabetes—Popular works. 2. Non-insulin-
    dependent diabetes—Treatment. I. Monk, Arlene. II. International
    Diabetes Center.
[RC662.18.M36 1995]
616.4'62—dc20   95-37503
                                                                CIP

CONTENTS

INTRODUCTION

Keeping your body healthy is a lot like keeping your car running smoothly. There are many parts within your body that rely on each other to function well. You need food for energy just as your car needs gasoline. And, though you hate to admit it, there is a timetable for maintenance for both your car and your body. Some people get their car's oil changed every 3,000 miles, while other people ignore it for as long as possible. Some people are very diligent about going to the doctor regularly, while others wait until a medical crisis. No matter what, sooner or later the car will need a maintenance check or repair work. Your body does, too. This is what managing your diabetes is about—improving your "routine maintenance" so that you can avoid the crises.

This book is about living healthfully and well when you, or someone you know, have type II diabetes. You may have heard type II diabetes described as "non-insulin dependent," "a touch of sugar," or "borderline diabetes." Or you may be under the impression that type II isn't the *serious* kind because you didn't get it as a child, or because you may not need to take insulin. But don't be misled—type II diabetes is a disease that needs careful attention in order to prevent or lessen damage to your body. However, managing type II diabetes is possible, and can in fact be done quite well! This book will teach you how.

Part One

TYPE II DIABETES AND YOU

A Brief History of Diabetes Mellitus

Ancient Egyptian writings (1500 B.C.) and later writings in Arabic and Chinese first described what we now know to be diabetes. The word "diabetes" comes from the Greek language and means "to flow through." "Mellitus" comes from the Latin language and means "honeyed." Therefore, our present-day term, diabetes mellitus, *aptly describes a condition in which there is sugar in the urine.*

Though ancient physicians could often diagnose diabetes, the medical outlook for the patient was bleak. Only in the last 200 years have we learned what causes diabetes and developed ways to treat it. In 1860, a German doctor named Paul Langerhans discovered clustered groups of cells in the pancreas that produce insulin. The discovery of these cells, which became known as the islets of Langerhans, paved the way for the experimental treatments that followed.

The big break in diabetes research came in 1921, when two researchers in Canada, Dr. Frederick Banting and Charles Best, discovered the beneficial effect of injecting insulin into dogs with diabetes. They then tried the treatment in humans, with nearly miraculous results. The discovery of insulin greatly improved the life expectancy of young people with diabetes.

Researchers soon discovered, however, that diabetes was not always caused by an absence of insulin in the body. They found that some people with diabetes had normal or even excessive amounts of insulin. These people had what came to be known as type II diabetes. And though type I and type II diabetes begin for different reasons, they are treated similarly.

Chapter 1

LEARNING ABOUT DIABETES

If you've just learned that you have type II diabetes, or if you are just learning how to take care of your diabetes, you're probably wondering how it's going to change your life.

It's not unusual to have many different thoughts and reactions about having type II diabetes. You may feel very worried and upset, or you may calmly conclude that you must not have the "bad" kind since you don't have any symptoms. You may believe that it was inevitable that you should get diabetes, since your family members had it. Or perhaps you have had type II diabetes for a long time and you'd like to learn more about it.

In this book you'll learn about many aspects of your health. Many of the guidelines for healthful living mentioned here are commonsense choices that everyone, whether they have diabetes or not, should strive to follow. You will also learn important information about diabetes, such as:

- what blood glucose (sugar) is and how to test for it;
- what the blood glucose test numbers mean;
- how food and activity affect your blood glucose;
- how to make food choices that are nutritious, balanced, and appropriate for maintaining blood glucose control;
- how to use exercise and physical activity to help control your diabetes and improve your health;
- what diabetes complications are and how to prevent them;
- how to cope with your feelings about having diabetes;

• how to identify roadblocks to change and make needed changes; and

• how to find the support you need to achieve your goals.

This may seem like a lot to learn, but knowledge is a powerful tool in helping you cope with your diabetes. The more you know about diabetes, the more effectively you can manage your care and live a well-balanced life. But before we get into the details of diabetes management, let's first look at what diabetes is.

What Is Diabetes?

When you have diabetes, your body cannot use food for energy very well. Much of the food you eat is digested and changed into glucose, a form of sugar. Glucose is the fuel your body needs for energy. When food is digested, the glucose enters your bloodstream and is carried to the cells in your body. A special substance is needed to help glucose enter your cells and be used for energy. That substance is *insulin*.

Insulin is a hormone that is made by your pancreas, a gland near your stomach. Insulin's job is to help the glucose in your bloodstream enter the cells. Insulin attaches to a specific location on the cell wall, called an *insulin receptor site*. From the insulin receptor site, the insulin tells the cell to take in glucose. The cell then uses the glucose for immediate energy or stores it to use later.

When the pancreas and insulin are working correctly, it's almost impossible for you to have too much or too little glucose in your

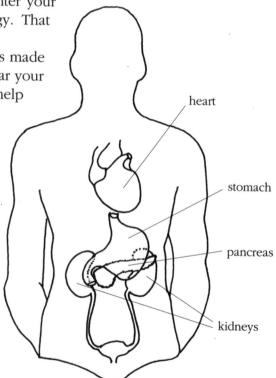

heart

stomach

pancreas

kidneys

Insulin is made in the pancreas

blood. When you eat, the pancreas responds by releasing the exact amount of insulin needed to help your body use the glucose from the food. Under these ideal conditions, your insulin supply is almost inexhaustible.

When you have diabetes, too much glucose stays in the bloodstream. This may be because the insulin-producing cells in your pancreas are making too little insulin. It may also be caused by too few insulin receptor sites on cells throughout your body. Or it could be because once the insulin attaches to the receptor site, its message or signal cannot get through to the cell. This makes you *insulin resistant*. Whatever the underlying cause, too much glucose stays in your bloodstream instead of going into your cells. The end result is a lack of energy. That's why you may feel tired when your blood glucose levels are high. However, diabetes develops gradually, and it is possible to have high blood glucose levels for long periods of time and not know it.

Your diabetes care will focus on your blood glucose levels because high blood glucose levels over time can cause a lot of damage to your body. Certain parts of your body are particularly sensitive to this problem, including your heart, blood vessels, feet, nerves, eyes, and kidneys. This is discussed further in Chapter 13.

Type II Diabetes

When you first develop type II diabetes the pancreas is producing insulin. But when the insulin is not working well, your pancreas knows it. Your pancreas senses the high glucose level in the blood and tries to make more and more insulin to help move the glucose into the cells. After years of overwork, the pancreas sometimes just wears out and cannot make enough insulin. If that happens, insulin injections are needed.

Scientists do not understand exactly why these problems occur. Studies suggest that some people inherit the tendency to develop type II diabetes. For these people, lack of exercise, stress, and extra weight somehow increase insulin resistance and can bring out type II diabetes. In many instances, exercising regularly, reducing stress, and making good food choices can help the body use insulin better and control blood glucose levels.

SYMPTOMS AND DIAGNOSIS. When your body does not use insulin as it should, your blood glucose levels go above the normal range. This glucose buildup can cause you to be very thirsty. You may need to urinate more frequently. Also, you may lose weight without trying. These are the classic or obvious signs of diabetes.

Some people may not have obvious signs, but instead have symptoms that do not immediately make them or their doctors think they have diabetes. These vague symptoms include feeling tired, being irritable, and having little or no energy to do things. Blurry vision, frequent infections, or pain, numbness, or tingling in the feet may be other signs. These kinds of problems sometimes mean that the person has had diabetes for some time.

Many times there are no early symptoms of type II diabetes and it is possible to have it for a long time without knowing it. Some people find out they have diabetes when they are being treated for another problem, like the flu or an infection. Other people may find out they have diabetes during a routine physical exam. Type II diabetes usually occurs in people over age 40.

If your health care provider thinks you have type II diabetes, one or two common laboratory blood tests can be done to verify whether or not you do. One is called a *random blood glucose*. For this test your blood is drawn and tested at any time in the day. If your blood glucose reading is 200 milligrams per deciliter (mg/dl, or 11.1 mM/L[1]) or higher, you would be diagnosed as having diabetes. A milligram is a small weight measurement. A deciliter is about three ounces of fluid.

The second laboratory blood test is called a *fasting blood glucose*. For this test you do not eat anything for 10 to 12 hours before blood is drawn. If your fasting blood glucose reading is 140 mg/dl (7.8 mM/L) or higher on at least two occasions, you are diagnosed as having diabetes.

TREATMENT. The treatment of diabetes is aimed at controlling blood glucose levels. You and your diabetes care team will decide what your initial treatment will be and what criteria you will use for changing treatments. To do this, you need to know what your treatment goals are and you need to have a time frame for meet-

---

[1] As a courtesy to readers outside of the United States, the millimole (mM/L) measurement is also listed. Note: mM/L x 18 = mg/dl.

ing those goals. If you follow your treatment plan and do not reach your goals within your time frame, you and your team can decide what your next step will be.

The methods of treatment usually proceed in a step-wise fashion. The first step in type II diabetes treatment is a healthful food plan and an exercise or activity program. Very often this alone can bring blood glucose levels down. Sometimes glucose-lowering pills or insulin injections are needed to treat type II diabetes. The goal is to keep your blood glucose levels as near to the normal range as possible. Testing your blood glucose regularly will let you know if you're reaching your goals. Two other goals are to keep your blood fats and blood pressure at healthy levels. Balancing the stress in your life can help a great deal with all of these aspects of your diabetes care.

Type II diabetes is a progressive disease. That means that it can do more and more damage to your body over time if you don't take care of it. It also means that anything you do at any time to care for your diabetes can help delay the progression. The most important thing to remember is this: Once you have type II diabetes, it will not go away—not even if you have no symptoms at all—and it is up to you to take control of your diabetes from the very first day.

Other Types of Diabetes

There are two other types of diabetes: Type I diabetes and gestational diabetes. These come about in very different ways from type II diabetes and are different from each other. Table 1.1 summarizes the three types of diabetes.

Type I diabetes is called insulin-dependent diabetes mellitus because people who have it must take insulin injections every day or they will die. In type I diabetes, the pancreas stops making insulin because the insulin-producing cells in the pancreas are destroyed by the person's immune system (auto-immune disease). You might know type I diabetes by its former name, juvenile-onset

---

[2] American Diabetes Association diagnostic criteria.

diabetes. It was called juvenile-onset diabetes because usually people younger than age 30 develop it. However, people of any age can develop type I diabetes.

It can be difficult to determine whether a person has type I or type II diabetes if he or she is diagnosed between ages 30 and 40. The classic symptoms can be similar in both types of diabetes. However, people with type I are often very thin and have large levels of ketones in their urine at diagnosis. Ketones are an acid by-product caused by burning too much fat for energy. People with type II are more likely to be overweight and usually have few or no ketones in their urine. It usually becomes clear in a short time if a person has type I diabetes because insulin injections are soon needed.

Gestational diabetes occurs when a pregnant woman's body cannot make enough insulin to accommodate the hormonal changes that occur naturally during pregnancy. Pregnant women need two to three times more insulin than usual to overcome these changes. All women should be tested for gestational diabetes between the 24th and 26th weeks of pregnancy.

The good news is that gestational diabetes is temporary and goes away after the baby is born.[3] However, women who have had gestational diabetes have a greater risk of developing type II diabetes later in their lives. The chances are greater if women are overweight before pregnancy or remain overweight after pregnancy. Proper eating habits, moderate exercise, and moderate weight loss can help women who have had gestational diabetes prevent type II diabetes.

Who Gets Type II?

Type II diabetes tends to run in families. Moreover, type II diabetes tends to run in American Indian, African American, Asian, and Hispanic families more frequently than in Caucasian families. The particulars of this genetic connection are not fully known, but the fact is that some of us are more likely to get type II diabetes than others.

---

[3] Occasionally gestational diabetes is actually type II diabetes that is discovered during pregnancy. In this instance, the woman will continue to have diabetes after the pregnancy ends.

TABLE 1.1 **Types of Diabetes**

QUESTION	TYPE I Insulin-Dependent Diabetes Mellitus (IDDM)	TYPE II Non-Insulin Dependent Diabetes Mellitus (NIDDM)	GESTATIONAL Gestational Diabetes Mellitus (GDM)
Who develops it?	Mostly children or adults under age 30, but it can happen at any age.	Mostly adults over 30 who have a family history of diabetes, are often overweight, and those of Hispanic, American Indian, African American, or Asian descent.	Two to five percent of pregnant women, usually during the second or third trimester (24–28 wks), those with a history of GDM, large infant, or family history of type II diabetes.
What are the symptoms?	Very thirsty, hungry, and tired. Need to urinate often. Unintentional, rapid weight loss. May have stomach pain and become very ill if not treated right away.	May not notice any symptoms or may have "vague" symptoms like tiredness, blurry vision, or frequent infections. May be thirsty and urinate often.	Symptoms are rare, may feel tired.
What is the cause?	The pancreas stops making insulin due to the destruction of the insulin-producing cells (called *beta cells*).	The body does not make enough insulin or cannot use its insulin correctly.	The hormonal changes of pregnancy demand more insulin than the body is able to produce.
Will it ever go away?	No	No	Yes, after the baby is born. However, the mother is at risk for developing type II diabetes later in life.
How is it controlled?	Daily injections of insulin, healthful diet, and exercise.	Healthful diet, exercise, and sometimes glucose-lowering pills or insulin injections.	Healthful diet, exercise, and sometimes insulin injections.

If you have diabetes, chances are good that you have a close relative who has diabetes too. Maybe you have seen firsthand how devastating diabetes can be. Maybe you've even had a relative die from diabetes or its complications. That can be frightening for you, for your children, and for other family members. It may even make you feel that the outcome of your diabetes is out of your hands or that you are doomed to the same fate. But that is not true.

There are many factors that determine the outcome of your diabetes. Likewise, there are many factors that you can change to improve your overall health. People with type II diabetes often have other health problems such as high blood pressure, abnormal blood fats, and obesity. These are often intertwined so that the steps you take to care for your diabetes may actually help not only your diabetes, but these other problems as well.

Living with Diabetes

The focus of this book is living *well* with diabetes. In fact, as you put your diabetes treatment plan into action, you may find yourself becoming and feeling healthier than you've ever been before. This is not uncommon. Almost one hundred years ago, Sir William Osler, a famous physician, remarked, "The way to live a long and healthy life is to have a chronic disease and take care of it." We hope that you will do just that.

Key Points

- When you have diabetes, your body can't use food for energy very well.

- Insulin helps glucose leave the bloodstream and enter the body's cells.

- There are three kinds of diabetes: Type I, type II, and gestational.

- Type II diabetes tends to run in families.

- Wise food choices and physical activity help improve blood glucose control and overall health.

Chapter 2

TARGETING YOUR CARE

Some people with type II diabetes think it is not as serious as type I diabetes because they may not need to inject insulin or may not have noticeable symptoms. Because of this thinking, they disregard advice from their diabetes care team about taking care of their diabetes. This chapter will explain why managing your diabetes is essential and how you can begin taking charge of your diabetes care.

Blood Glucose Levels

As mentioned in Chapter 1, much of your diabetes care will focus on your blood glucose levels. To better understand what blood glucose levels and numbers mean, let's first look at people who do not have diabetes. Their blood glucose levels stay in a very narrow range. After fasting all night or before meals, their blood glucose is usually between 70 and 115 mg/dl (3.9 and 6.4 mM/L).

Even right after eating, people who do not have diabetes have a blood glucose level that rarely goes above 140 mg/dl (7.8 mM/L). This means that their bodies respond to glucose in their bloodstreams by releasing the right amounts of insulin. The glucose is helped into the cells by insulin and then used for energy or stored for future use.

Everyone's blood glucose levels go up and down throughout the day. Your blood glucose levels are affected by the foods you eat, how active you are, the medicines you take, and how relaxed or stressed you are. The main way you can control your blood glucose level is to keep all these things in balance.

Your Target Blood Glucose Range

The primary goal of diabetes care is to keep your blood glucose levels as close to the normal range as possible. However, it may not be realistic to expect your levels to be normal 100 percent of the time. Therefore, people with diabetes have *target blood glucose ranges*—a span of numbers to stay within. The target range identifies where you would like your blood glucose level to be most of the time. Table 2.1 shows normal blood glucose ranges and suggested ranges for people with diabetes. Your diabetes care team will help you decide on the target range most appropriate for you. Make sure all team members agree on the target range so that you are all working toward the same goals.

In order to know what your blood glucose levels are, you will need to test your blood. This is called self blood glucose monitoring or SBGM. SBGM is a simple test that you do to measure your blood glucose at certain times of the day. You and your team will decide what times of the day and how often you will test your blood glucose. A member of your diabetes care team can teach you how to test. It is also explained in Chapter 8.

By keeping track of your blood glucose levels at different times of the day, you can learn how your blood glucose is affected by food, physical activity, and diabetes medications if you take any. You can then adjust what you eat, drink, and do in order to keep your blood glucose at healthful levels. As a result, you will feel better on a daily basis and lower your chances of developing diabetes-related problems.

When blood glucose levels are too high, it is called *hyperglycemia*. "Hyper" means "high." When you have high blood glu-

TABLE 2.1 Blood Glucose Ranges

Time of Day	Normal	Target in Diabetes
Fasting or before meals	70-115 mg/dl (3.8-6.4 mM/L)	80-140 mg/dl (4.4-7.8 mM/L)
1-2 hours after meals	Below 140 mg/dl (7.8 mM/L)	100-180 mg/dl (5.5-10 mM/L)

cose levels, you may feel extra thirsty and tired and need to urinate more often than usual. These are the same symptoms many people have when they are first diagnosed with diabetes. However, you may not notice any symptoms with hyperglycemia, so testing your blood glucose regularly is very important.

If a person's blood glucose gets too low, it is called *hypoglycemia*. "Hypo" means "low." The signs of hypoglycemia include feeling shaky, dizzy, sweaty, sleepy, or confused. However, not everyone has symptoms when their blood glucose level is low. Testing your blood glucose is the only way to know for sure.

Blood Fats (Lipids)

Another important goal of diabetes care is to control the levels of fats (triglycerides and cholesterol) in your blood. High cholesterol and triglyceride levels can lead to serious health problems, including heart disease and stroke. Blood fats can be controlled by the same things that help control your blood glucose levels—making wise food choices and staying active. It is important for you to understand what blood fats are and to know what your levels are, so you can make changes in your eating habits and activity level if necessary.

CHOLESTEROL. Cholesterol is a waxy substance found in foods that come from animals. Your liver also produces cholesterol to help make hormones, bile acids, and strong cell walls. Some people's bodies naturally make more cholesterol than others do, and this tends to run in families. If this is true in your family, you can't change your genetic tendency, but you *can* alter your lifestyle by increasing your activity and choosing low-fat foods. Reducing the amount of fat you eat—especially saturated fat—is a critical step toward reducing your cholesterol levels. Limiting your intake of meats, organ meats, eggs, and fat-containing milk products will help reduce your cholesterol too. A healthy total blood cholesterol level is under 200 mg/dl (5.2 mM/L).

Cholesterol does not dissolve in the blood, so it must be carried through the bloodstream by a protein. There are three main types of proteins that carry cholesterol, and these are called lipoproteins. "Lipo" means "fat." Each lipoprotein has a specific purpose.

13

Low-density lipoprotein (LDL) cholesterol carries cholesterol in the bloodstream and is often called the "bad" cholesterol. When there is too much LDL-cholesterol in the blood, it combines with other substances to form deposits on the blood vessel walls. This causes a narrowing of the blood vessels and increases the risk of heart disease. A healthy LDL-cholesterol level in someone with diabetes is less than 130 mg/dl (3.35 mM/L), and less than 100 mg/dl (2.58 mM/L) if you have heart disease.

High-density lipoprotein (HDL) cholesterol is often called the "good" cholesterol. A high level of HDL-cholesterol protects against heart disease. It removes cholesterol from the blood vessel walls and carries it back to the liver to be disposed of. HDL-cholesterol is not affected by what you eat but can be raised by regular exercise or weight loss. A healthy HDL-cholesterol level is 35 mg/dl (.9 mM/L) or higher for men and 45 mg/dl (1.16 mM/L) or higher for women.

Very-low-density lipoprotein (VLDL) cholesterol is the major carrier of triglycerides to the fat cells for storage.

TRIGLYCERIDES. Triglycerides are a combination of three fatty acids and are the fats found in foods. Some fat you eat is absorbed and transferred to your fat cells as triglycerides. Insulin allows triglycerides to enter the fat cells for storage. People with diabetes may have high triglyceride levels because the insulin in their bodies cannot complete this process. The triglycerides stay in the bloodstream which can lead to heart disease. A healthy blood triglyceride level is less than 200 mg/dl (1.56 mM/L), or less than 150 mg/dl (1.17 mM/L) if you have a history of heart disease.

Following your food plan is the most important thing you can do to help lower your blood cholesterol and triglyceride levels and keep them under control. You will be working on a food plan in Chapter 9. Also, Chapter 14 gives guidelines for when to have your cholesterol and triglycerides tested.

A Treatment Plan for You

Your treatment plan is set up based on your lifestyle and health care needs. It will include eating a balanced diet, being physically active, and monitoring your blood glucose levels. Your plan may also include daily doses of pills to treat your diabetes (also called glucose-lowering pills or oral agents) or insulin injections. The goal of your treatment plan is to keep your blood glucose levels within your target range most of the time.

FOOD AND EXERCISE. Every treatment plan for people with type II diabetes includes guidelines for eating healthful foods and increasing physical activity. Of course, good eating and exercise habits are important for all people, whether or not they have diabetes. But for you, these two things are even more important because they help control your blood glucose levels.

As we've discussed, food is changed to glucose, which is carried in the blood to all parts of your body. Food makes blood glucose levels go up. Physical activity makes blood glucose levels go down. Food and activity need to be balanced in order to keep your blood glucose levels in your target range.

With the help of your diabetes care team, you can create a treatment plan that outlines what, how much, and how often to eat and what kind of activities to do. This plan can be tailored to fit your personal interests and needs. For example, your dietitian can help you create a food plan that suits your schedule, tastes, and budget. Your doctor, diabetes educator, or exercise specialist can help you choose activities that are safe for you and that you enjoy.

GLUCOSE-LOWERING PILLS AND INSULIN. Another part of your treatment plan may be to take glucose-lowering pills or to inject insulin. The pills help your body produce more insulin or better use the insulin it already makes. Insulin injections add more insulin to your system so that your body is better able to use glucose for energy.

If your doctor prescribes glucose-lowering pills or insulin injections, it does not mean your diabetes is "worse." It just means that your body needs pills or insulin as well as a healthful diet and regular exercise to control your blood glucose levels. If your blood glucose levels stabilize due to both medications and new food and activity habits, it is possible that you may need to take pills or insulin for only a short period of time.

Your treatment plan is not a "fixed" program. You may need to make changes from time to time depending upon how your body responds to different treatments and what your blood glucose levels are. You and your diabetes care team will work closely to make sure that your treatment plan is working.

Setting Goals and Getting Started

As with many other challenges in life, it's easier to manage your diabetes when you deal with it one day at a time. Remember, you did not get diabetes overnight, and you do not have to master it overnight.

The first place to start is to schedule regular visits with your doctor and other diabetes care team members. The list of who your team members may be is on page 160. They can help you set diabetes care goals and help you evaluate how you are doing. But remember, you are the most important member of the team.

Key Points

- The goal of diabetes treatment is to keep your blood glucose levels as close to normal as possible.

- Blood glucose levels are affected by the foods you eat, how active you are, the medicines you take, and how relaxed or stressed you are.

- People with diabetes have individual target blood glucose ranges that identify where they would like most of their blood glucose readings to be.

- Self blood glucose monitoring (SBGM) is a simple test you use to measure your blood glucose level.

- When blood glucose levels are too high it is called *hyperglycemia.* When blood glucose levels are too low it is called *hypoglycemia.*

- An additional goal of treating type II diabetes is to keep blood fats (lipids) under control.

- A treatment plan for type II diabetes includes a food plan, exercise and, if necessary, glucose-lowering pills or insulin.

Chapter 3

LIVING WITH DIABETES

Each year, over 500,000 people are told, "You have type II diabetes." And because they are unique people, they react to this news in very different ways. A 38-year-old writer may be afraid that eye problems will steal her livelihood. A 72-year-old retiree may worry that the daily care of diabetes will be too much for him, and that he will lose his independence. Some are relieved that it isn't something worse and immediately start learning ways to manage their diabetes. More often, people find it hard to embrace a chronic illness that demands constant self-care and raises the possibility of long-term complications. Many people feel angry and frustrated. Others decide to deal with diabetes by ignoring it and waiting until something "really" goes wrong.

Whether your reaction is like one of these or something different, one fact remains sure—people have an emotional response to diabetes. The feelings you experience after you are diagnosed are not "good" or "bad." They are a natural part of grieving for your healthy self—the self you knew before you had diabetes—and of adjusting to your new circumstances. And people *do* adjust. For some it takes longer than others, and the emotional paths people travel can be very different.

Learning to identify what emotions you are feeling is a vital part of adjusting to diabetes. The following statements and explanations are examples of common ways people respond to diabetes. You may, of course, experience thoughts and feelings that are not included here, and you may feel many emotions at the same time. This overview is intended only as a starting point to help you begin to identify and think about your own feelings.

Emotional Reactions to Diabetes

> *"I don't have to change."*
>
> *"I don't have to control my diabetes."*
>
> *"If I stop thinking about diabetes, it will go away."*
>
> *"I know that I should be (testing my blood, following a food plan, exercising) but I ignore it all."*

DENIAL

Some people would rather not deal with having diabetes. Life was easier before they knew they had it, so they pretend it's not there. They are in a state of denial. Denial is not a feeling. Rather, it is a way of stopping feelings from coming to the surface. Denial often serves as a self-protection mechanism when someone feels too much stress or pain. Sooner or later, the feelings push their way out. Much of the time feelings come back even stronger when you "stuff" them.

Eventually, when you're ready, you need to deal with diabetes and the feelings you have because of it. If you deny that you have diabetes, you will not take care of yourself as you should. And after years of neglecting your diabetes, you could develop serious health problems. Diabetes will not go away, even if you ignore it.

> *"What's going to happen to me?"*
>
> *"I'm worried about making mistakes with my food plan, blood testing, or exercise."*
>
> *"When people talk about complications, I don't listen."*
>
> *"I don't test when I think my blood glucose result will be high."*

FEAR

The fear people have about diabetes comes from some very real concerns. Type II diabetes is a serious disease that can have many complications. Perhaps you already have numbness in your feet, an infection that won't heal, or a toe or foot amputation. These are difficult and frightening health problems. You may feel as if you've lost control of your body. You may fear that you won't be able to adhere to a food plan because you've always had trouble eating what you should or keeping your weight down. Feelings of lack of control or fear of failure are common. It's good to recognize and acknowledge these feelings. Anytime there is change in our lives, we tend to respond by feeling fear.

To an extent, fear serves a good purpose. It can prompt you to seek the information you need to control your diabetes. A reasonable level of fear can motivate you to take care of yourself. It may prompt you to talk to your spouse, friend, clergyman, or doctor about your fears. On the other hand, too much fear over a long period of time can lead to a feeling of hopelessness. It can cripple you by taking the joy out of your life. Usually your fear will lessen as you gain knowledge about your diabetes and regain control of your health by following a treatment plan. If you feel overwhelmed with fear, seek help from a counselor as soon as possible.

ANGER

Anger is a natural reaction to the unwanted, unexpected, and undeserved diagnosis of type II diabetes. It is also a powerful emotion that is uncomfortable to face. Accept that it's okay to feel angry for awhile following your diagnosis, or at

"It just isn't fair!"

"I'm being cheated by diabetes."

"I often snap at my family, friends, and care team."

different times when diabetes seems to get in the way of your life. In moderate amounts, anger is healthy and normal. It can give you the energy you need to deal with your health concerns. Think of it as just one part of adapting to your new circumstances.

Anger becomes unhealthy when you feel it too strongly for too long, or when it's directed in a harmful way. For example, you may feel tempted to take your anger out on the people around you. Or you may take your anger out on yourself by not following your doctor's advice. In such cases it's best to talk it out with a trusted friend or counselor.

GUILT

You may feel guilty if you believe you have done something wrong or have caused yourself to get diabetes. Too much guilt is harmful. If you feel guilty all the time, you may start to believe that you're "bad" or a "failure." Instead of taking better care of yourself, you are more likely to neglect your health.

"If I just hadn't eaten so much sugar."

"I did something bad and now diabetes is my punishment."

"I'm afraid to report my food habits and my blood test numbers because I'll be judged as a bad person."

However, feelings of guilt can be useful and beneficial, too. These feelings serve as a reminder to us to live as responsibly as

19

we can. You may need a little guilt to get you back on track with your treatment, such as following a food plan, increasing your activity level, or testing your blood glucose regularly.

SADNESS

"I feel so alone; no one understands what I'm going through."

"I cry all the time."

"I feel hopeless."

Sadness is a normal response to being unable to change a situation you don't like. You probably will spend some time denying your diabetes or feeling fear, guilt, or anger as a first reaction. The sadness comes once you realize that diabetes will not go away.

Feeling sad is an important stage in the process of adjusting to life with diabetes. During the time you are sad, you will begin to make some necessary changes in your self-image to include diabetes. You will focus on how diabetes will affect you and what your life will be like from now on. Feeling sad is one more step in the process of adapting to the reality that you have diabetes.

Sadness can develop into depression if it lasts too long. Signs of depression are loss of energy, decreased appetite, sleeping problems, and feelings of hopelessness. Depression is a serious problem that can be treated with counseling and sometimes medication. If you begin to feel overwhelmed by sadness, tell a friend, family member, or counselor as soon as possible. There is help available.

FRUSTRATION

"I'll never be able to get my blood glucose under control."

"I want to talk about my diabetes with friends, but they don't want to listen."

"I try hard to manage my diabetes, but sometimes it doesn't make any difference."

You may feel frustrated when you're learning how to manage your blood glucose levels. Oftentimes glucose levels fluctuate from day to day, even if you eat and do the exact same things as you did the day before. Managing your diabetes is sometimes "easier said than done."

Extreme frustration can lead to anger and some of the feelings described earlier. When you feel frustrated, try to step back and look at the situation calmly and realistically. Recognize the aspects of your care that are going well

"I'm for real"

Now that my e-mail includes my company name,
I look more professional. Customers notice.

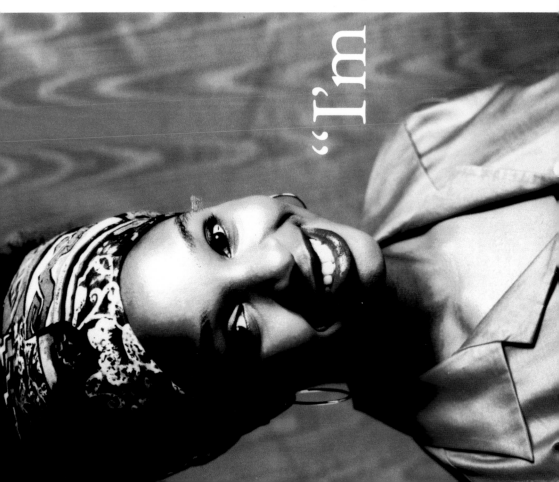

Get your
personalized e-mail address — and get down to business.

- Enhance your image
- Promote your business
- Reach customers easily

With VeriSign it's:

- **Smart** — Advertise your business with every e-mail you send.

- **Essential** — Check e-mail from anywhere, via any Web browser. Works with Outlook, Eudora and other programs. Includes e-mail address and matching domain name.

- **Easy** — It takes only minutes to set up your e-mail — just point and click.

  Plus get 24/7 customer support from the company with over 5 million customers on the Web.

Go to www.myverisignmail.com
to get your personalized e-mail address

Reply by September 20!

Limited Time Offer

Save **33%**

When you register for 3 years — that's less than $33 a year.*

Hurry — reply by September 20!

A22

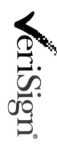

VeriSign Processing Center
1730 M Street NW, Suite 700
Washington, DC 20036

Is it available? Search free to find out.
trudy@my-own-company.com

Ms. Trudy K. Smith
1012 W. Lincoln Ave.
Goshen, IN 46526-2127

and congratulate yourself for them. If you have trouble dealing with your frustration, talk it over with someone you trust.

RELIEF

Perhaps you expected worse news than "you have diabetes." You then felt relieved when you learned you have diabetes because it's a manageable disease. On the other hand, maybe your relief made you relax and think diabetes isn't very serious. That isn't true. Controlling your blood glucose levels will go a long way toward preventing diabetes complications. You'll feel healthier too.

> "Thank goodness. I can handle this."
>
> "It could have been worse!"
>
> "I have a friend with diabetes, and she's doing okay."

HOPE

Feelings of hope can sustain you even when you feel anxious about the future. The strength you gain from hopeful feelings can "put the spring in your step" and help you face any challenges that come your way.

> "Scientists will find a cure for diabetes in my lifetime."
>
> "I take care of my diabetes the best I can each day."
>
> "I keep up-to-date on new advances in treating diabetes."

ADAPTATION

With time and effort, you can learn to adapt to diabetes. You will start to feel better physically in a short time if you follow your diabetes care team's advice. It may take you longer to feel better emotionally, however.

> "I can cope with having diabetes."
>
> "I don't like watching what I eat, but I understand why it's important."
>
> "I will learn everything I can about diabetes."

You can learn to live well with diabetes through reaching a kind of balance in your life. This balance encompasses making some lifestyle changes and starting to see diabetes as a part of you. Take heart in knowing that reaching this balance is not a neat, orderly, and predictable process. At times everything will fall into place and at other times you may feel overwhelmed. Do not be surprised if you feel fear, anger, or sadness all over again. You will probably cycle through various emotions many times as you live with diabetes.

Diabetes and Your Family

Having diabetes affects both you and the people close to you—your spouse, children, parents, and friends. They, too, need time to adjust to diabetes. They may go through some of the same feelings that you do—they may be relieved that it wasn't something worse, for example, or they may fear that you will develop complications. Your family may also need time to adjust to your treatment schedule. Some of the changes you need to make in your routine, such as eating at regular times, will affect them too.

Though they may need time to adjust, your family can play a big part in supporting you and helping you cope. It's important to educate them about diabetes—what it is, what lifestyle changes you will have to make, and how they should handle diabetic emergencies.

Take family members along to visits with your diabetes care team or to diabetes education classes. Talk to your family about specific ways they can give you support as you care for yourself each day. You may ask, for example, that they eat healthful meals with you, or go on walks with you a few times a week. If you often forget to test your blood glucose or take your medication, ask for their help in remembering.

Seeking Support

Family members are not the only people who can provide support during rough times. You may not have family members close by, or you may need more support than your family and diabetes care team can give. If you find yourself in one of these situations, seek out a counselor or clergy member in whom you can confide.

If sometimes you feel like you're the only one in the world with diabetes, consider joining a support group. Support groups are safe places where people with diabetes can talk about their feelings and listen to others who may be experiencing similar concerns. Members can also share good things that have happened in their lives, and discuss possible solutions to problems that they've encountered with their diabetes.

If you decide to look for support from a counselor or group, ask your diabetes care team if they know of existing resources in your area (see also Resources on page 179). Asking for help may be a new step for you, but it's an essential one. The isolation you may experience if you don't have a support network can affect how you care for your diabetes. It is important for you to take control of the situation and get what you need. No one will do it for you, and you will benefit greatly from the support you receive.

Coping with Stress

Adjusting to diabetes emotionally goes beyond your initial response to the news that you have diabetes. Living with a chronic illness that involves lifestyle changes, a complex schedule of medical care, and potential complications creates a whole range of ongoing stresses. Coping with diabetes means learning to balance these stresses, along with the normal pressures of daily life, so that you feel good emotionally and physically. In Chapter 6, we will look at strategies for managing stress.

Key Points

- Some of the emotions you may feel about your diabetes include denial, fear, anger, sadness, frustration, relief, hope, and adaptation.

- When family members find out that you have diabetes, they may go through an adjustment similar to yours.

- Friends, family members, counselors, support groups, or clergy members can all be sources of emotional support.

Part Two

THE BASICS OF DIABETES CARE

You're Not Alone:
The Demographics of Diabetes

How Many People Have Diabetes?

It is estimated that about 16 million people in the United States have some form of diabetes. Of those people, nearly half do not know they have diabetes and therefore are not receiving care for it. Each year, between 500,000 and 700,000 people are diagnosed with diabetes.

Who Gets Type II Diabetes?

The most common form of diabetes is type II (non-insulin dependent diabetes mellitus). This form usually develops in adults over age 40 and is most common in adults over age 55. In the U.S. population ages 65 to 74, nearly 17 percent of whites have diabetes, 25 percent of blacks have diabetes, and 33 percent of Hispanics have diabetes. Slightly more women than men tend to get diabetes, particularly among blacks. American Indians have the highest rates of diabetes in the world. In one tribe, the Pima Indians, half of all adults have type II diabetes.

Who Gets Type I Diabetes?

About 800,000 people in the United States have type I diabetes (insulin-dependent diabetes mellitus). Girls are usually diagnosed with diabetes between ages 10 and 12, and for boys the peak time is between ages 12 and 14. Type I diabetes occurs equally among males and females, and it is more common in the white, non-Hispanic population. Some northern European countries, including Finland and Sweden, have very high rates of type I diabetes.

Sources: American Medical Association, U.S. Department of Health and Human Services, and American Diabetes Association

Chapter 4

EATING WISELY, EATING WELL

Nutrition is the number-one way of managing type II diabetes. It is often called the "cornerstone" of diabetes care because eating wisely and well is a must for good blood glucose control and for good health. The goals of nutrition in diabetes care are:

- to keep your blood glucose levels as close to normal as possible;
- to achieve healthy levels of blood fats (lipids);
- to help you reach and maintain a reasonable weight; and
- to meet your nutrition needs.

The things you can do to achieve these goals are shown in Figure 4.1. Factors such as food choices, the timing of meals, and the amount of food eaten all affect your ability to control your blood glucose levels. In short, if you want to keep your blood glucose levels in your target range and meet your nutrition needs, then you need to pay attention to what, when, and how much you eat.

The notion of watching *what* and *how much* food you eat is probably not new to you. In fact, it may sound suspiciously like a diet. But for people with diabetes, the impact of this idea reaches far beyond that of a diet. This is because certain foods affect your blood glucose level more than others. The more you eat of foods that raise your blood glucose, the harder it may be for you to control your blood glucose levels.

Interestingly, the recommendations for what and how much to eat that you will learn about in this book are the same recom-

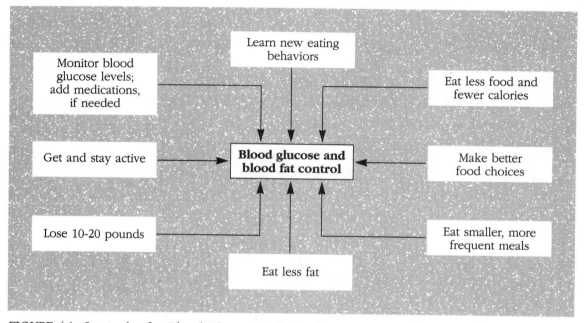

FIGURE 4.1 **Strategies for Blood Glucose and Blood Fat Control**
Adapted from *Maximizing the Role of Nutrition in Diabetes Management,* © 1994, with permission from American Diabetes Association

mendations suggested for everyone, whether they have diabetes or not. It is just good nutrition. Watching what and how much you eat can also help you reach and maintain a reasonable weight.

Considering *when* you eat probably is a new idea. The reason the timing of meals and snacks is important in diabetes is because you are trying to match the food you eat with the insulin available for using the food. If you eat more food at one sitting than your body's insulin can handle, the glucose from the food stays in your bloodstream, causing high blood glucose levels. On the other hand, skipping or delaying meals or snacks can cause your blood glucose level to go too low, especially if you take insulin.

Spacing meals and snacks throughout the day, as well as eating smaller amounts of food at each meal and snack, can help keep your blood glucose levels from going too high after eating. It also helps control your appetite while giving your body energy throughout the day—the time when you are most active.

Part of your diabetes treatment is following a food plan that details what, when, and how much you should eat. This is not as strict or as unpleasant as it sounds. Your food plan is a guideline, not a set diet. And you will be surprised at the flexibility you have in your meal planning and food choices. You will learn more about this when you work on your own food plan in Chapter 9. For now, let's look at what makes up the food we eat so we can understand why good nutrition, good food choices, and a food plan are so important in diabetes treatment.

Food Nutrients

There are six nutrients in food, and each has a special role in our bodies. The nutrients are carbohydrate, protein, fat, vitamins, minerals, and water. The first three—carbohydrate, protein, and fat—give our bodies energy or fuel, which is measured in calories. Each of these nutrients needs insulin to be used correctly. The last three—vitamins, minerals, and water—help regulate our body processes and do not contain calories or need insulin to be used. We will focus on carbohydrate, protein, and fat since these nutrients require insulin to be used properly.

CARBOHYDRATE. Carbohydrate is a very important nutrient in nutrition and in diabetes care. It is the body's first choice for energy or fuel, and it is the nutrient that has the greatest effect on blood glucose levels. Carbohydrate is found in a variety of foods that seem unrelated, such as bread and grains, milk, fruit, and vegetables. Carbohydrate is also found in table sugar and foods that contain sugars.

All carbohydrate, no matter what the source, can raise your blood glucose if you eat too much at one time. But don't think you have to avoid carbohydrate foods. Carbohydrate foods are a very important part of good nutrition. Your food plan will give guidelines for how much carbohydrate to eat at meals and snacks. Spacing your carbohydrate foods throughout the day helps to control your blood glucose levels. You will also learn by experience how to adjust the amount of carbohydrate foods you eat based on your blood glucose test results.

PROTEIN. Protein is found in many foods, including meat, fish, poultry, cheese, eggs, milk, dried beans, peas and lentils, nuts,

TABLE 4.1 **Nutrients Used for Energy**

NUTRIENT	FUNCTION	SOME FOOD SOURCES
Carbohydrate	The body's first choice for energy or fuel. Carbohydrates affect your blood glucose the most.	
	Sugars (naturally occurring and added) are an energy source. They are also carbohydrate in its simplest form.	*Naturally occurring:* Fruits, vegetables, and milk *Added:* Table sugar, honey, soft drinks, syrup, candies, pies, cakes, cookies, jams, and jellies
	Starches are made up of many sugars that are linked together in long chains.	Breads, cereals, pastas, grains, rice, and starchy vegetables, such as potatoes, corn, peas, lima beans, and squash
	Fiber is the "structure" in some foods. It is not digested by the body, and it helps the body remove waste.	Whole-grain breads and cereals, fruits, vegetables, and legumes (dried beans, peas, and lentils)
Protein	Essential for forming new tissue, repairing damaged tissue, and maintaining muscle, skin, and blood health. Some can also be changed into glucose for energy.	Meat, fish, poultry, cheese, eggs, milk, dried beans, peas, lentils, nuts, and seeds
Fat *10% or less of daily intake should be from saturated fats*	A concentrated energy source that provides essential fatty acids for normal body function. Fat is the body's second energy source.	
	Polyunsaturated and *monounsaturated fats* are liquid at room temperature and help lower blood cholesterol levels.	Most vegetable oils such as olive, canola, peanut, corn, cottonseed, safflower, soybean, sunflower; olives, peanuts, and walnuts
	Saturated fats are solid at room temperature and raise blood cholesterol levels.	Butter, cheese, meats, lard, palm oil, coconut oil, cocoa butter, and solid vegetable shortenings

and seeds. Protein from these foods is digested and enters the bloodstream as *amino acids*. With the help of insulin, these amino acids are used to form new tissue or to repair tissue. People with diabetes who do not have enough insulin in their bodies may have slow-healing wounds because the amino acids cannot be used properly. Amino acids the body gets from protein can also be changed into glucose for energy or into fat for future energy.

Protein foods have little effect on blood glucose. However, many protein foods, like meat, contain fat. Choosing foods wisely and controlling portion sizes will assure that you get the protein you need without also eating too much fat.

FAT. The fat in food supplies a concentrated form of energy that is needed for proper body function. Fats also carry vitamins A, D, E, and K, which are important for good nutrition. Fat is present in meats, margarines, oils, salad dressings, many dairy products, many snack and prepared foods, and desserts.

There are three main kinds of fat: saturated, polyunsaturated, and monounsaturated. Usually, all are present in those foods that contain fat. The fat that is present in the largest amount determines what the food is called. Monounsaturated or polyunsaturated fats are preferable to saturated fat because saturated fats can raise your blood cholesterol levels and increase your risk for heart problems.

Fat does not raise blood glucose levels. However, eating large amounts of fat can interfere with the body's ability to use insulin and can make it more difficult to control blood glucose levels. It can also contribute to weight gain, heart disease, and other health problems. Having diabetes means you are already at risk for these health problems. It is important to control the fat in your diet so that you don't add to your risk. Table 4.1 on page 30 summarizes the functions of carbohydrate, protein, and fat in our bodies and gives examples of foods that contain each.

Food Nutrients and Insulin

When you have diabetes, the way your body uses food nutrients is directly related to how well your body is using insulin. Insulin helps your body use carbohydrates, protein, and fat for energy and nutrition. When enough insulin is present and it is working well,

"Let Me Eat Cake!"

Traditionally, people with diabetes were told to avoid table sugar and foods with added sugar because scientists believed sugar raised blood glucose levels higher and faster than starches. Research has shown, however, that a carbohydrate is a carbohydrate whether it's a starch or a sugar. Equal amounts of starch or sugar have the same effect on blood glucose.

Can you eat a small piece of cake, a cookie, or another sugar-containing dessert if you have diabetes? Usually yes, but you need to know how to substitute that food for another carbohydrate food in your food plan. The key is to keep your carbohydrate intake consistent, so you shouldn't just add the dessert on top of what you would normally eat. Occasionally, you may decide to eat a cookie or a small piece of cake *in place of* a fruit or starch. Just be sure to check the serving size so the carbohydrate content of the cake closely matches what you would have gotten from the fruit or starch.

Generally, dessert portions will be small because they are a concentrated source of sugar and usually contain a lot of fat and calories. Managing your diabetes is easier if you limit yourself to no more than one small dessert per day.

the food you eat is used for energy, building strong tissues, normal healing, and future energy stores. If your body does not have enough insulin or is not using it correctly, the result is high blood glucose levels, lack of energy, poor healing, high blood fat levels, and difficult weight loss. This is illustrated in Figure 4.2.

Eating small meals and snacks spaced throughout the day allows the insulin in your body to work better and helps keep your blood glucose levels from going too high or too low. You will especially want to distribute the carbohydrate foods you eat among your meals and snacks so you don't overload your system with too much glucose at one time. This also helps assure that you have enough glucose available when your body needs it.

The Food Guide Pyramid

A good way to learn about how to eat for better blood glucose control is to study the Food Guide Pyramid. The pyramid was developed by the U. S. Department of Agriculture (USDA) to reflect current nutrition guidelines. It shows foods divided into six groups and gives the number of servings to eat each day for good nutrition. You've probably seen the pyramid on food labels or in your grocery store.

The pyramid shown in Figure 4.3 is adapted from the Food Guide Pyramid to better reflect the needs of people with diabetes. Let's now look at the different levels of the pyramid.

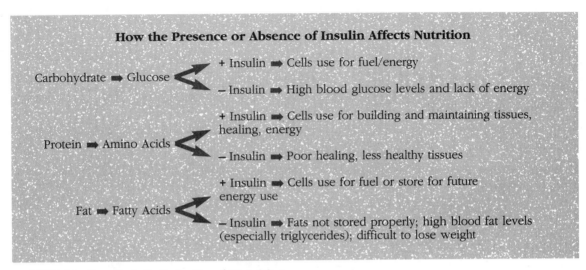

How the Presence or Absence of Insulin Affects Nutrition

Carbohydrate ➡ Glucose

+ Insulin ➡ Cells use for fuel/energy

– Insulin ➡ High blood glucose levels and lack of energy

Protein ➡ Amino Acids

+ Insulin ➡ Cells use for building and maintaining tissues, healing, energy

– Insulin ➡ Poor healing, less healthy tissues

Fat ➡ Fatty Acids

+ Insulin ➡ Cells use for fuel or store for future energy use

– Insulin ➡ Fats not stored properly; high blood fat levels (especially triglycerides); difficult to lose weight

FIGURE 4.2 **Insulin's Role in Good Nutrition**

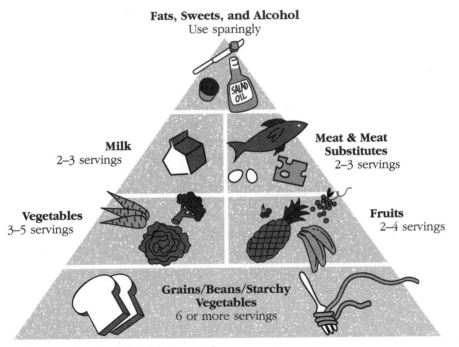

FIGURE 4.3 **Food Guide Pyramid**
Adapted from *Food Guide Pyramid*, © 1994, U.S. Department of Agriculture

The bottom level of the pyramid shows foods that are the foundation of good nutrition. Most of these foods are made from grains. Starchy vegetables such as potatoes, corn, and squash are included in this group because the nutrients they supply are similar to foods made from grains. For the same reason, dried beans are also included in this group. Foods from this group are a major source of carbohydrate and will play a big part in your food plan. One serving of a food from this group supplies 15 grams of carbohydrate and is called one *carbohydrate choice*. Choose six or more servings from this group each day.

The second level of the pyramid contains fruits and vegetables. Eating fruits and vegetables adds important vitamins, minerals, and fiber to your diet. Vegetables (except the starchy types on the bottom level) are low in carbohydrate and calories and can be eaten liberally. Choose three to five servings a day. Fruit does supply a significant amount of carbohydrate. One fruit serving is one carbohydrate choice (15 grams of carbohydrate). Choose two to four fruit servings a day.

The foods in the third level of the pyramid are necessary for the protein, calcium, iron, and zinc they provide. One milk serving provides 12 to 15 grams of carbohydrate and is one carbohydrate choice. Though cheese may seem to be more like milk than meat, it is included with the meat group because it does not contain carbohydrate and does not have the same effect on your blood glucose as milk and yogurt do. One meat, poultry, fish, or cheese serving is two to three ounces (one-half whole chicken breast or one leg and thigh, a serving of meat about the size of a deck of cards, or one medium fish fillet). Choose two to three milk servings and two to three meat servings each day.

The foods at the top of the pyramid give you calories and not much else, so choose them sparingly and eat small amounts.

Remember that foods from all the food groups are essential for well-balanced, good nutrition. But serving sizes are just as important as food choices. This is true for everyone, not just people with diabetes. We often forget that when we eat twice the amount of a food, we are eating twice the calories and nutrients too. Learning and understanding serving sizes is essential to good nutrition. As a person with diabetes, your special emphasis will be on when you eat, as well as what and how much, to help keep your blood glucose in your target range.

Diabetes and Weight Loss

The main goal of your diabetes treatment is to achieve blood glucose control—not to lose weight. However, reaching and maintaining a reasonable weight can help with blood glucose control, as the diagram below illustrates. Research studies show that people who lose even a modest amount of weight, between ten and twenty pounds, often see an improvement in their blood glucose levels. Other health benefits of weight loss include better blood pressure control and healthier blood fat levels.

If you have type II diabetes and are overweight, you are not the only one; many people with type II diabetes struggle with this problem. Also, many factors may be working against your efforts to lose weight. Your family history, body structure, activity level, age, and other health factors can affect your body weight and your ability to lose weight.

Weight loss

Cells lose their resistance to insulin

Cells become sensitive to insulin so body uses insulin better
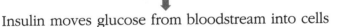
Insulin moves glucose from bloodstream into cells

Cells use glucose
↓
Blood glucose levels begin to return to normal

People with type II diabetes often are "insulin resistant" as well. This means that over a period of time cells in the body become resistant to the action of insulin and do not use insulin effectively. Excess body fat, especially abdominal fat around the waist, can contribute to this insulin resistance which, in turn, contributes to high blood glucose levels. Moderate weight loss can decrease insulin resistance and help you keep your levels within your target range.

Sometimes, losing weight means you can lower your dose or stop taking glucose-lowering pills or insulin injections. If your blood glucose tests show levels at or below the low end of your target range, or if you need to eat more to keep your blood glucose levels from going too low, you probably need to adjust your medication. If any of these things happens to you, discuss changing your dose with your diabetes care team.

Key Points

- The goals of nutrition in diabetes are to help you control your blood glucose and blood fat levels, stay at a reasonable weight, and eat a healthful diet. There are a number of strategies you can use to meet these goals.
- Insulin is needed by the body in order for it to use carbohydrate, protein, and fat for energy and nutrition.
- Carbohydrate has the greatest effect on your blood glucose level.
- The Food Guide Pyramid can help you learn how to make healthful food choices each day.
- Losing ten to twenty pounds can help improve your blood glucose and blood fat levels.

Chapter 5

GETTING ACTIVE, STAYING ACTIVE

No advice about health and well-being is more often received with groans of protest than the advice to start exercising. Nor is there any other advice that, if taken, can so dramatically *improve* your health and well-being. This is a simple fact that is true for all people. However, when you have diabetes, exercise is not only advisable, it is an integral part of your diabetes care.

For most of us, the word "exercise" conjures up images of people huffing and puffing through an exercise class, or of well-conditioned, tireless athletes breezing past us on the jogging path. You may think that exercise has to be hard to be good, or that you need to have special physical attributes to do it. But recent research shows that even moderate physical activities like walking and yard work—things we all do every day—have many of the same health benefits as traditional exercise.

Physical activity is any movement that uses energy. *Exercise* can be thought of as more vigorous physical activity. We are all physically active, some of us more than others. But no matter where you are on the physical activity scale, you can start now to

How active are you?
Mark the spot on the physical activity scale.

| Very Sedentary | Sedentary | Somewhat Active | Moderately Active | Extremely Active |

improve or maintain your activity level. Anything you do—whether it's walking around the block or playing three sets of tennis—will help improve your health and your diabetes control.

Health Benefits of Physical Activity

It's hard to imagine anything more beneficial to health than physical activity. It makes you stronger and more flexible. It helps tone your muscles and "burn" fat or calories and it helps you to control and maintain a reasonable weight. Physical activity keeps your heart and blood vessels in shape so blood and oxygen are more efficiently transported throughout the body. It also can make you feel better by giving you an outlet for stress and increasing your energy.

These benefits reduce your risk of atherosclerosis, high blood pressure, and heart disease, health problems which are all too common in our population today. They are even more common in people with diabetes. It's important for you to be aware that increasing your physical activity by even a small amount can make a big difference in your diabetes management and your general health.

One of the most important effects of increased physical activity on health is that it decreases cholesterol and triglycerides in the blood. Cholesterol and triglycerides are the two major "blood fats" or fatty material in your blood. High cholesterol and triglycerides can lead to heart problems. Physical activity decreases the triglycerides and "bad" LDL cholesterol in your blood while it increases the levels of "good" HDL cholesterol. There is nothing better you can do for your heart health.

The Activity Advantage . . .

- *For every hour of physical activity, another hour—or more—may be added to your lifetime.*

- *Sedentary people are twice as likely to develop heart disease than those who are more physically active.*

- *High blood pressure occurs twice as often in inactive people as in active people.*

- *Even moderate activities cause the body to burn more calories from fat and help to control weight.*

- *Many people report greater self confidence, increased productivity, and less stress, anxiety, and depression after becoming more active.*

Physical Activity and Blood Glucose Control

In addition to improving your overall health, physical activity helps you keep your blood glucose levels in your target range. While excessive amounts of food can cause your blood glucose level to rise, activity causes it to go down. Much of your diabetes treatment is focused on balancing food and activity in your daily life. The better balanced the two are, the better your blood glucose control will be.

Activity lowers blood glucose levels in two ways. First, it causes your cells to become more sensitive to insulin. This means your insulin actually works better and more glucose is used by the cells. This sensitivity to insulin and the benefit of lower blood glucose levels lasts for several hours, even after activity has ended.

The second way that physical activity lowers blood glucose is by lowering the amount of glucose produced in the liver. Besides getting glucose from the food you eat, you also get glucose from your liver. Although producing glucose is a normal function of the liver, it sometimes makes more glucose than your body can use, causing your blood glucose level to go up. Regular activity as part of a healthy lifestyle can help counter this effect.

Physical activity will help you get and keep your blood glucose in control. The effects of increased activity are so great that some people are able to decrease their diabetes medications or even stop taking them altogether. But even if this doesn't happen, the benefits of better glucose control, better health, and more energy are well worth the investment.

Getting and Staying Active

Most of us know physical activity and exercise are good for us, but most of us still don't do it. If you find it hard to start and stick to an exercise program, take heart. You are not alone. It is estimated that only 20 to 30 percent of adults participate in regular physical activity. One reason for this may be the furor with which the exercise movement swept over us in the 1970s and 1980s. We were told that we had to exercise 30 to 40 minutes at "high intensity" at least three or four times a week. When we couldn't go out and "just do it," we became discouraged and "just gave up" instead.

It is said that in youth we learn and in age we understand. Now that the exercise movement is middle-aged, we are getting wiser about what our bodies need to be healthy. Thankfully, moderation has won out. Experts now believe that exercising for 10 minutes three times a day can be as beneficial as exercising continuously for 30 minutes. The repetitious jarring of the jogging track and the wild abandon of high-intensity aerobics classes are not the only ways to a healthier you.

The moderate approach to activity and exercise suggests that you have to start where you are. If you have been inactive, begin by making small changes in your daily habits to increase your activity level. Use the stairs instead of the elevator, park at a distance and walk to a store's entrance, do yard work, or stand and stretch during the day to get your body moving and your blood flowing. Allow yourself to start slowly and to increase your activity level gradually. The goal is to become a more active person overall in your life—not necessarily to follow a set exercise routine week after week. If you have been sporadically active, try to make physical activity a regular part of your life. Of course, if you are very active, keep it up.

Becoming active is the first step, but staying active is equally important. The health benefits of physical activity begin to disappear after only three days of inactivity. And if weeks or months go by with no activity, you may need to start again at a lower level than you had been used to. Consistency is the key to the long-term benefits of physical activity, so start slowly and take it at your own pace. Trying to do too much too soon can cause you to become discouraged and it may be hard to keep at it.

In Chapter 11 you will have a chance to develop a personal physical activity plan. The important thing to remember is that any physical activity will benefit your health and your diabetes control.

The Activity Pyramid

You have already learned about the Food Guide Pyramid and how it can help you choose a nutritious and healthful diet. The Activity Pyramid has been developed to help you become a more active person. It shows how you can build variety and enjoyment into your active lifestyle.

The foundation of physical activity in our lives is formed by the things we do as we move through a typical day. We work, we run errands, we take care of our children and our homes. For some of us—perhaps those who have small children or have physically demanding jobs—daily life can be naturally very active. This used to be true for almost everyone before cars and automation moved our society away from agriculture and toward industry. But today, most of us need to think about ways we can be more active during our daily lives. The bottom level of the pyramid represents our daily activity and suggests ways we can increase it.

The next two levels of the pyramid show a variety of activities that can really help you improve your physical fitness. The aerobic activities strengthen your heart and lungs, while flexibility and strength activities improve muscle tone. Recreational and leisure activities help to round out an active life. These types of activities usually need to be planned and very often can be more enjoyable when shared with one or more exercise partners.

The top level of the pyramid represents the inactive time in your day. We all need some time to sit and relax. The problem is that most of us do too much sitting. Because computers, television, and office jobs are so prevalent in our world, it is easy to set-

CUT DOWN ON
Sitting for more than
30 minutes at a time
Watching TV
Playing cards
Knitting

Leisure
Golf
Bowling
Gardening

2–3 TIMES A WEEK

Flexibility and Strength
Weightlifting
Stretching
Yoga
Tai Chi

Aerobic Exercise
Brisk walking
Running
Bicycling
Swimming
Cross-country
skiing

3–5 TIMES A WEEK

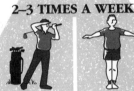

Recreational
Tennis
Dancing
Hiking

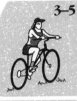

EVERY DAY
Walk the dog
Take longer routes
Take the stairs instead of the elevator
Walk to the store or mailbox
Park your car farther away
Make extra steps in your day

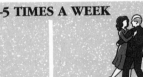

FIGURE 5.1 **Activity Pyramid**
Adapted from *The Activity Pyramid,* © 1995 Institute for Research and Education
HealthSystem Minnesota

Tips to Help You Become More Active

Visualize. See yourself as a person who feels good, looks good, and has energy. Think positively about yourself and your body.

Work through excuses. Look for ways to overcome your usual excuses for not being active. For example, if your excuse is that you are just too tired to do anything after work, go for a 20-minute walk at lunchtime instead.

Be prepared to make sacrifices. You need to devote time to your activity, and you'll have to make decisions and set priorities. You might have to miss (or videotape) your favorite TV show if it conflicts with your exercise time.

Establish goals and rewards. Think of short-term, intermediate, and long-term activity goals and reward yourself when you reach them. Think of something that motivates you, then work to give it to yourself!

Find a partner. Activities and exercise are often more fun when you have someone to share them with. Also, a partner can help you stick to your program. Ask a friend, a neighbor, a spouse, or another family member to join you. Or find a class. Even an exercise video can be a motivator.

Build in variety. Find several activities, indoor and outdoor, to participate in. Boredom can set in quickly if you do the same thing all the time. You might swim on Monday, do an exercise video on Wednesday, and walk on Saturday. Fit in some housework and gardening during the week and you'll be in good shape in no time.

Plan for your activities. Set aside time during the day for exercise. Many people find it helpful to schedule an exercise "appointment" in their daily calendar. Make exercise a priority so the time doesn't get used for something else.

Make it fun. If it's not fun, you probably won't do it. Find the activities and exercises you enjoy and figure out how to make it as much fun as possible. Exercise should not feel like work. It's more like a gift you give yourself.

WEDNESDAY
- 8 -

11:45 - Walk at Lunch

tle into an inactive life. Just as we need to think about ways to be more active every day, we need to be conscious of how much time we spend sitting. Most of us can do with less.

Remember, there is more to an active life than exercise classes or running. You will do best if you can look at the whole of your life and try to make it as active as possible. That's how the Activity Pyramid differs from the Food Guide Pyramid. With activity, more is better!

If You Have Health Problems

Moderate physical activity is safe for most people, but there are some risks you should be aware of. When you know what the risks are, you can avoid injury and problems while having a great time getting fit.

The complications of diabetes are a special concern when you are starting a program of physical activity. These include heart disease, high blood pressure, neuropathy, and retinopathy. If you have any of these complications, consult with your doctor or diabetes care team before you begin an exercise program.

HEART DISEASE OR HIGH BLOOD PRESSURE. Strenuous exercise often can be more harmful than helpful when you have heart disease or high blood pressure that is not controlled by medications. Your doctor or diabetes care team can help you select a level of activity that will help keep your blood pressure from going too high. When you do begin exercising, you should watch for any signs of trouble, such as shortness of breath; extreme tiredness; dizziness or faintness; or chest, shoulder, or arm pain. If you notice any of these signs, stop your activity immediately. Before you exercise again, tell your doctor about your symptoms. If you have a history of heart disease, a cardiac stress test may be helpful so that you and your doctor can determine the level of intensity you should work toward.

NEUROPATHY. If you have nerve damage (neuropathy), you may not be able to feel pain in the affected area or your balance may be slightly off. When you have these concerns, avoid exercises that could injure your hands or feet (volleyball, soccer, hockey) or that rely too much on your arms and legs for support (walking, aerobics, standing exercises). Seated activities like the armchair aerobics discussed in Chapter 11 are a good choice for people with neuropathy. Always wear well-fitting and supportive shoes and socks, and check your feet after you exercise to look for blisters or reddened areas. Treat any injuries appropriately.

Some neuropathies (autonomic neuropathy) make it hard to feel chest pains that could signal a heart attack. If you have this concern, talk to your diabetes care team to learn which activities are safe for you.

RETINOPATHY. If you have eye disease related to your diabetes (retinopathy), you need to do activities that will not raise your blood pressure too much. High blood pressure can make your retinopathy worse. Always stay within the activity level that is comfortable for you. If you are breathing very heavily, slow down. Your activity should not cause you to breath very heavily or pant, and you should never hold your breath during the activity. If you have retinopathy or have had recent laser eye surgery, avoid activities that cause you to bounce, jump, or strain.

Almost everyone can be active and safe if they make the right choices and use a little caution. You will learn about the many activity choices you have and create a personal activity program that's right for you in Chapter 11. So get ready to get fit and have fun!

Ask Your Doctor . . .

Talk to your doctor before you begin an exercise program if you:

- *are over age 40 and are not exercising regularly;*
- *have had type II diabetes for 10 or more years;*
- *have uncontrolled high blood pressure;*
- *have heart trouble, heart murmur, heart attack, or a family history of heart disease before age 55;*
- *feel pain or pressure in any area of your body during mild activities;*
- *have bone or joint problems;*
- *experience shakiness, dizziness, sweating, faintness, blurry vision, or headaches;*
- *have had high blood glucose levels for several months;*
- *have low blood glucose levels—lows for several weeks or several lows per week; or*
- *have shortness of breath or breathlessness after mild activity.*

Key Points

- Physical activity is any movement that uses energy. Exercise can be thought of as more vigorous physical activity.
- Physical activity is an important part of your treatment plan because it helps control your blood glucose levels.
- Exercise can help reduce your risk of artherosclerosis, high blood pressure, and heart disease.
- Physical activity does not have to be strenuous to be beneficial.
- There are many activities from which to choose, so there is something for everyone!
- To achieve lasting benefits from physical activity, it is important to be consistent in your activity.

Chapter 6

BALANCING STRESS

Everyone knows what it is to feel stress—the pounding heart, the clammy hands, the adrenaline rush. You can probably name a dozen things in daily life that trigger your "fight or flight" response. And it's not just the angry bosses, crying toddlers, and traffic jams of the world that cause us stress. Even the events that we normally consider positive—marriage, family gatherings, getting a promotion—can be stressful.

It would be impossible to eliminate stress from our lives, since stress is another way of describing our responsiveness to life. As Canadian stress expert Dr. Hans Selye said, "The person without any stress—is dead." Moreover, banishing stress entirely would not even be desirable. Manageable levels of stress can create useful energy, stimulate our creative abilities, and challenge us to solve problems.

But too much stress can harm a person's emotional and physical health. And for people with diabetes, stress can make blood glucose levels difficult to control. This means that it's especially important for you to find sound strategies for managing stress.

Stress and Diabetes

As you probably know, diabetes can add stress to your life. Monitoring your blood glucose, making sure you eat and exercise on time, and taking medications can sometimes be time-consuming and irritating. Your diabetes care schedule does not always mesh well with schedules of family members, co-workers, and the rest of the world.

It also works the other way around; stress can affect diabetes. The major hormones involved in a stress reaction—adrenalin, noradrenalin, glucagon, cortisol, and growth hormone—cause the blood glucose level to rise. People who don't have diabetes produce insulin to balance this blood glucose elevation. But in people with diabetes, the actions of these stress hormones may contribute to poor blood glucose control. This is not universal, however; some people experience lower blood glucose levels when they are under stress.

The best way to find out how stress affects your diabetes is the personal scientist approach: when you're stressed, test your blood glucose level to see what happens.

Stressful times may be the very times you don't want to bother with taking good care of your diabetes. But because stress can change your blood glucose level, you especially need to take care of your diabetes when you're under stress. This means that during stressful times, it's important to:

- eat healthfully;
- exercise regularly; and
- stay on your schedule of blood glucose monitoring and medications.

Eating well and exercising not only help you keep your blood glucose under control, they can help relieve stress as well. It's also important to find other healthy ways to manage stress in order to keep your blood glucose—and your life—in balance.

External and Internal Stressors

Before we can begin to manage the stress in our lives, we must first identify the situations that cause it. While our specific stressors may seem countless, they all fall into one of two categories: external stressors and internal stressors.

External stressors come from outside ourselves. These include both major stressful events and minor, everyday irritants. Think about those things in your life that cause stress for you, such as conflicts with family members or co-workers, financial worries, traffic, too much to do in too little time, and so on. Just having diabetes can add stress to your life. Identifying your daily hassles and conflicts is an important first step in discovering what you can do to manage stress.

Internal stressors come from inside us. Generally people are less aware of these stressors, but they're likely to play an even greater role in the creation of stress in daily life. Let's look at some examples of internal stressors.

VALUES AND BELIEFS. These are deeply held philosophies we usually learn in childhood and hold to be absolute. They can be very positive, helping to direct our lives. But when people around us do not share our beliefs, we can feel stress. We can also feel stress when events in our lives force us to reevaluate what we believe and value.

FAITH. Our faith can be extremely valuable in helping us cope with life's challenges. It can also be a source of internal stress, particularly if we believe we should be perfect and able to adhere to all the doctrines of our faith without exception. Because we are human, we may find we are not living according to our professed beliefs. This discrepancy is a significant source of internal stress, creating guilt and perhaps a sense of failure. To address this discrepancy, we must change either our belief or our behavior. We might recognize that we can adhere to our faith and yet be human, modifying our expectations. Or, if our expectations are already reasonable, we might change our behavior so that it is more in agreement with what we actually believe.

GOALS. As children, many of us were taught to "shoot for the moon." Our parents naturally like to instill a sense of confidence in us, and this confidence can help us set and achieve many of our goals. But sometimes it can lead us to establish goals that are unrealistic. Having overly high expectations sets us up for failure and, therefore, a great deal of internal stress. When we miss targets, we focus on what we have *not* achieved rather than what we have accomplished. Feelings of failure become not only a source of internal stress, but an obstacle to further effort.

Setting realistic, achievable goals for success is the real motivator. When you accomplish goals, you affirm your capability and motivate yourself to try for new goals. If you happen to have a goal that is too high to reach immediately, break it into smaller steps so you may experience the sense of success that will motivate your continued efforts.

SELF-CONCEPT. We all have an image of who we are mentally, physically, socially, and spiritually, and we constantly evaluate that image. People used to think that if you talked to yourself you were crazy. Now we know that we talk to ourselves all the time. We have an internal monologue in which we evaluate ourselves and everything around us. Often this monologue and our self-evaluations come from comments about us or responses we have received over the years. Unfortunately, we often tend to minimize the positive feedback from others and magnify the negative or critical comments. This leaves us with an internal voice that's often negative and self-critical: "I never do anything quite right." "I'm worthless, I'm a failure, I don't deserve anything good." These "killer phrases" erode self-esteem and make people less happy, less effective, and less likely to take care of themselves. The problem with this kind of thinking is that it adds a great deal of internal stress and may become a self-fulfilling prophesy.

Listen to your internal voice. If you hear those killer phrases, catch yourself. Make these negative statements more realistic and balanced by adding a positive side: "I may not be perfect, but I have many strengths and abilities." Think of your accomplishments and of qualities you like about yourself, and work them into your internal monologue. And when others pay you compliments and give you affirmations, remember them if you start to feel down about yourself. Changing the negative cycle does not happen overnight. But once you begin to talk to yourself in more encouraging ways, you'll begin to live up to your positive expectations.

Errors in Thinking

Errors in thinking often occur when an external stressor and an internal one collide. An external hassle or difficulty arises, and we make the situation more stressful by viewing it irrationally. The following examples show thought patterns that add unnecessary stress to our lives.

ALL-OR-NOTHING THINKING. This type of black-or-white thinking is evident in statements such as, "If I don't follow my diabetes schedule perfectly, there is no point in doing it at all." The problem is that few things in life are black or white. In this example, it definitely *is* better to follow your diabetes schedule, even if you don't do it perfectly. All-or-nothing thinking sets up unrealistic expectations because it's nearly impossible to "do it all." To lessen the stress caused by this type of thinking, try to look at the "gray" zone and begin to set more realistic expectations.

MAGNIFICATION. Magnification occurs when we overestimate the importance of a negative event or overreact to it. A person may see one high blood glucose reading and panic, thinking "something terrible must be happening." Magnification can often be identified by words such as "awful, horrible, or terrible." While these words are appropriate in some situations, we often use them in situations where they don't belong, such as being late, spilling something, getting stuck in traffic, or being criticized. When you find yourself thinking this way, ask yourself if those words are appropriate, or if you need to put the problem in perspective.

"SHOULD" STATEMENTS. We often try to motivate ourselves with "shoulds" or "oughts," believing that if we tell ourselves often enough that we should do something, we'll do it. In reality, we just build up an enormous list of what we believe are our obligations, and we become overwhelmed. We're left with a lengthy list of "shoulds" and no action. This discrepancy can be a significant source of internal stress.

Instead of drowning yourself in "shoulds" and "oughts," choose one thing you would like to accomplish, perhaps the one that's most important to you. Make sure it's realistic, then change the way you say it. Instead of "I should do...," say "I choose to do..." or "I will do...." Changing "shoulds" to "choose to" or "will" can help you turn the procrastination and excuses into action.

Strategies for Balancing Stress

There are many ways we can cope with the stress in our lives—talking to a friend or counselor, writing in a journal, taking a bubble bath, even watching a football game. But in general, there are two ways you can respond to a stressful situation. You can try to *change the situation* in order to reduce or eliminate your stress. Or you can try to *change the way you think and feel* about a stressful situation—you can look at the problem in a way that causes less stress. In some situations, it's helpful to use both strategies.

CHANGING THE SITUATION. Suppose you're trying to stick to your food plan, but your spouse is always keeping sweets around the house. This makes trying to eat healthfully even more difficult for you, and you're starting to feel resentful of your partner's freedom to eat less nutritious foods. In this situation, you can take action to change the stressful situation. You can sit down with your partner and explain how important it is for you to eat healthful foods and how difficult this becomes with so many sweets around. You might ask your partner to eat healthier food with you at home and save the junk food for other times and places. Or you might find another solution that works for both of you.

When you're in the middle of a stressful situation, making changes can seem impossible. Try to step back from a stressful situation and identify which aspects you can realistically change. Then try to brainstorm, alone or with a friend, a number of alternatives. The changes you consider may be large—for example, you may choose to leave a pressure-cooker job for a more flexible one—but they may also be necessary for your health and well-being. Often you may find smaller ways to alter a situation so that stress is not overwhelming.

CHANGING HOW YOU THINK AND FEEL. Many situations that cause us stress—having diabetes, for example—can't be changed. They are simply part of our lives, and we need to find ways to cope with them. Following are some suggestions for ways that you can begin to view them in a more positive way.

Broaden the way you think about stressful situations. Often we dwell too long on the negative aspects of a stressful situation. We tell ourselves we can't handle it, we blow the situation out of proportion, and we miss opportunities for personal growth. While we can't eliminate all the negative feelings we have when we're under stress (these feelings are natural and can even be helpful), we *can* view the situation in positive ways as well.

Search for ways to turn stressful situations into positive ones. Look at a conflict with a co-worker as an opportunity to improve your interpersonal skills. Or if you're stressed because you can't stick to your exercise program, try to find an opportunity in it. For instance, you might take family members along on your walks and use the time to talk and build your relationships. Every problem you face is an opportunity to gain experience and wisdom.

Learn to relax. Methods of inducing relaxation such as yoga, meditation, deep breathing, and biofeedback are different techniques with the same goals. They help to change your body chemistry, release your muscular tension, and focus your mind on something other than your problems. Relaxation techniques give your body a release from tension and your overtaxed brain a break from worrying. When you're relaxed, you can approach your stressors in a calm manner and with an open mind. Ask your diabetes care team if they know of local counselors, therapists, or other specialists who can teach you about these techniques. Your local community education program (call your school district) or community center may also offer classes in relaxation.

Seek support. When you feel burdened by stress, one of the most helpful things you can do is confide in someone you trust and with whom you feel comfortable. Most of us confide in our friends, spouses, and co-workers when we have something to get off our chests. Much of the time, this is enough.

Sometimes, however, your level of stress may become so great that you need more help than those people close to you can offer. In cases like this, consider speaking with a counselor. A counselor can help you work through particular problems you are experiencing, and may be able to help you view stressors in a new, less stressful way. A counselor also can help you decide if you want to take action to change a stressful situation. He or she may be able to teach you relaxation techniques to help you get through routine stresses that pile up. If you don't know of a good counselor, ask a close friend, clergy member, or member of your diabetes care team to recommend one.

The Balancing Stress Pyramid

The strategies listed previously can help you deal with specific stresses as they arise. But it's also important to develop habits that help you cope with the "hassles" of daily life. The Balancing Stress Pyramid lists ways you can keep daily stress at a manageable level by balancing the stressors in your life with small things you do to take care of yourself.

The bottom level of the pyramid is the foundation for meeting

DANGER ZONE
Overeating
Over drinking
Withdrawing from others
Negative self-talk
Depression

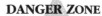

Hobbies   **2–3 TIMES A WEEK**   **Rewards**
Reading   Bubble bath
Gardening   Massage
Woodworking   Dinner out
Golf   Buy something new
Sewing

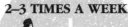

Relationships   **3–5 TIMES A WEEK**   **Grounding**
Seek support   Attend religious services
Family time   Meditate
Socialize   Spend time alone
Communicate feelings   Write in journal

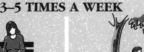
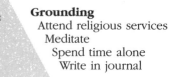

EVERY DAY
Healthful eating & enough sleep
Physical activity
Fulfilling work or hobby
Positive self-talk
Positive interaction with others
Laughter & hugs

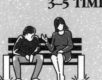

FIGURE 6.1 **Balancing Stress Pyramid**
© 1995 Institute for Research and Education HealthSystem Minnesota

the challenges of daily life. Note that some of the basic requirements for good physical health—healthful eating, physical activity, and adequate sleep—are also part of a sound stress-management strategy. Physical activity, in particular, is a wonderful outlet for pent-up stress. At the foundation, too, are the things that make daily life enjoyable and worthwhile such as laughing and talking with others and working at a fulfilling job or hobby.

The second level of the pyramid represents our sense of self, our relationships with other people, and our spirituality. Confiding in another person is often a good way to cope when you feel sad or anxious. Even when we're not under extreme stress, we need to nurture our relationships. Just as important is time to ourselves, to relax and think about our values and dreams, and to think about our lives in a "big picture" kind of way.

The third level of the pyramid represents the special ways that we can be kind to ourselves. It's surprising to realize how easy it is to forget or ignore our own needs as we try to meet the demands of life. Work, family, friends—all are important, but they can't always come first. Take the time to notice what you need and give it to yourself. Even a small gift to yourself can do a lot to lift your spirits.

The top level of the pyramid shows the danger zone, which can be the result of unbalanced or unhealthy stress. When stress becomes overwhelming, people often find themselves involved in negative behaviors as a way of seeking relief. Think of the ways you behave when you're under too much stress. Be aware that some of these behaviors may be dangerous to your health and well-being. Also, you may be tempted to ignore your diabetes care. If you find that you cannot control your unhealthy behaviors, seek help from a friend or counselor.

As you can see, there are a variety of ways to manage the stress in your life. Different stressors demand different approaches, and some techniques may work better for you than others. Explore different strategies and find out what works for you. And don't get stressed out about managing your stress—just set realistic goals for adding stress management techniques to your life, and take it from there. Remember, you don't have to do it alone. Family, friends, your diabetes care team, support groups, and mental health professionals are all a part of the support network that can help you manage your stress.

Key Points

- Both positive and negative events can cause stress.
- For people with diabetes, stress can make blood glucose levels more difficult to control.
- It's important to take especially good care of your diabetes during stressful times.
- There are two types of stressors: external (from outside ourselves) and internal (from within ourselves).
- Stress may result from errors of thinking—from viewing ourselves or our problems irrationally.
- We can respond to a stressor either by changing something about the stressful situation, by changing how we feel or think about the situation, or by doing both.
- It's important to balance the everyday stressors in life with things you do to take care of yourself.

Chapter 7

TREATING DIABETES WITH MEDICATIONS

A combination of healthful eating and physical activity is the key to diabetes care and good health, so the first step in treating type II diabetes is usually a food and activity plan. These alone can occasionally get blood glucose levels within the target range, and some people do well on this treatment for years. However, when eating well and staying active do not result in reaching and maintaining blood glucose goals, other treatment options must be considered.

Glucose-lowering pills are used *with* a food and activity plan to enhance diabetes treatment when blood glucose goals are not being met. The medication *does not replace* a food and activity plan. Glucose-lowering pills are also called diabetes pills, oral hypoglycemic agents, or just oral agents. They are typically taken once or twice a day.

If glucose-lowering pills do not bring blood glucose levels within the target range, insulin may be prescribed. Insulin is taken by injection one to four times a day, depending on blood glucose patterns and goals. Again, the food and activity plan continues after insulin injections are added.

The fact that you need medication (glucose-lowering pills or insulin injections) to control your blood glucose levels does not mean that you did anything wrong. Each individual responds to treatments differently. These steps in diabetes treatment reflect *your* options for treating *your* diabetes. The important thing is to focus on whatever you must do to reach and maintain your blood glucose goals.

Glucose-lowering Pills

Different types of glucose-lowering pills help lower blood glucose levels in one or more of the following ways:

- The pancreas is stimulated to release more insulin.
- The body's cells become more sensitive to insulin.
- The release of glucose by the liver is decreased.
- The body absorbs glucose from food more slowly.

Three types of glucose-lowering pills are currently available in the United States to treat diabetes: *sulfonylureas, biguanides,* and *alpha glucosidase inhibitors.* Sulfonylureas work primarily by stimulating the pancreas to release more insulin. Biguanides work by decreasing the release of glucose by the liver and by making cells more sensitive to insulin. Alpha glucosidase inhibitors slow the body's absorption of carbohydrates. These medications may also be used in combination, since each lowers blood glucose in a different way.

Sulfonylureas have been used for years to treat diabetes. Both "first generation" and "second generation" sulfonylureas are available. In the pharmaceutical industry, "generation" refers to the course of drug development. Later generations are usually considered to be improvements of some of the drug's properties. However, this doesn't always mean that they are better for *everyone* than an earlier generation. Second generation sulfonylureas are used in smaller doses, have fewer interactions with other drugs, and may have fewer side effects than first generation sulfonylureas.

Biguanides have been used in other parts of the world for many years, but only recently has one been approved for use in the United States. It is called metformin (Glucophage®). The potential advantages of metformin are that it can minimize or eliminate the hypoglycemia and weight gain that are often associated with sulfonylureas. Also, metformin tends to reduce levels of blood fats (cholesterol and triglycerides), which are often high in people with type II diabetes.

Alpha glucosidase inhibitors are taken before each meal and delay the body's absorption of carbohydrates. An alpha glucosidase inhibitor called acarbose (Precose®) was recently approved for use in the United States.

Once it is decided that glucose-lowering pills are needed, any of these three medications may be prescribed. Different pills are taken in different daily doses and act for different periods of time. Your doctor will work with you to find the one that best suits your needs and effectively lowers your blood glucose. Table 7.1 lists the glucose-lowering pills currently available in the United States, along with common starting doses.

Your blood glucose test results will help you and your doctor decide on a starting dose that is right for you. It may be higher or lower than the dose listed in Table 7.1. Expect to increase your dose every one to two weeks if your blood glucose levels do not improve. The dose can be increased until the maximum dose per day is reached, unless you experience side effects. Your doctor may decide to use a combination of different glucose-lowering pills as you work toward your target blood glucose goals.

Some glucose-lowering pills may cause your blood glucose levels to go too low. If this happens, your dose may be decreased.

TABLE 7.1 **Glucose-lowering Pills**

Trade Name	Generic Name	Common Starting Dose	Maximum Dose/Day	Schedule
Second Generation Sulfonylureas (More commonly used)				
DiaBeta®	glyburide	1.25–5.0 mg	20 mg	1–2 times daily
Micronase®	glyburide	1.25–5.0 mg	20 mg	1–2 times daily
Glynase®	glyburide (micronized)	1.5–3.0 mg	12 mg	1–2 times daily
Glucotrol®	glipizide	5.0 mg	40 mg	1–2 times daily
Glucotrol XL™	glipizide (extended release)	5.0 mg	20 mg	1 time daily
First Generation Sulfonylureas (Less commonly used)				
Orinase®	tolbutamide	500–1000 mg	3000 mg	2–3 times daily
Diabinese®	chlorpropamide	100–250 mg	750 mg	1 time daily
Dymelor®	acetohexamide	250–500 mg	1500 mg	1–2 times daily
Tolinase®	tolazamide	100–250 mg	1000 mg	1–2 times daily
Biguanides				
Glucophage®	metformin	500–1000 mg	2550 mg	1–3 times daily
Alpha glucosidase inhibitors				
Precose®	acarbose	50 mg	300 mg	3 times daily

Occasionally people are taken off glucose-lowering pills if their blood glucose levels are too low on the lowest dose of medication.

PRECAUTIONS. Glucose-lowering pills cannot be used by certain people. People with type I diabetes and women who are pregnant or breast-feeding should not take these medications. People who are allergic to sulfa drugs should discuss this with their doctor before starting a sulfonylurea, since these drugs can share some common side effects. People with liver or kidney disease may not be able to use glucose-lowering pills, because their bodies may not be able to break down and excrete the medication effectively. If this happens, the medication can build up in the body, causing severe hypoglycemia or other dangerous side effects.

Glucose-lowering pills should not be used if you:

- *are pregnant;*
- *are breast-feeding;*
- *have kidney or liver disease;*
- *have type I diabetes (though Precose® may sometimes be used in combination with insulin);*
- *have other serious medical problems (seek medical guidance from your doctor); or*
- *drink excessive amounts of alcohol.*

POSSIBLE SIDE EFFECTS. As with any medication, glucose-lowering pills may cause some side effects. These problems do not happen very often, but you should be aware of what could happen. In rare instances, people may notice a rash, hives, or fever. If you have any of these symptoms or if you notice other changes in your body after you begin taking any medications, stop taking the medication and tell your doctor. You may be having an allergic reaction to the medication.

The most common side effect of the sulfonylurea medications is *hypoglycemia* (low blood glucose). Since these pills stimulate the pancreas to make more insulin, which in turn lowers your blood glucose level, it is possible that your blood glucose will go down too much. This can happen when meals are delayed or skipped or when the medication dose is too high. Symptoms of hypoglycemia include feeling shaky, sweaty, tired, hungry, dizzy, crabby, or confused. When you have any of these symptoms, test your blood glucose if you can. If it is low, eat a food with carbohydrate (such as four ounces of fruit juice or one cup of milk) to bring your blood glucose level back up into your target range. If you can't test and you feel any of these symptoms, eat a food with carbohydrate. You can read more about hypoglycemia and how to treat it on page 78.

Whenever you experience hypoglycemia, it's important to try to understand why it happened. Think about when and what you last ate, and your activity level during the few hours prior to your symptoms. If you can't figure out why your blood glucose got so low, call your doctor. You should also call your doctor if you have symptoms of hypoglycemia more than two times in a week. It may be that your medication dose needs to be lowered.

The most common side effect of biguanide medications (metformin)—and rarely seen with sulfonylureas—is gastrointestinal upset. Symptoms include diarrhea, nausea, or vomiting. If you notice heavy breathing, shortness of breath, extreme fatigue, sleepiness, dizziness, or disorientation, stop your diabetes medication and call your doctor immediately. These can be signs of *lactic acidosis,* a condition seen rarely in people taking metformin.

Alpha glucosidase inhibitors such as acarbose can also cause gastrointestinal symptoms such as cramping, gas, and diarrhea. These symptoms usually pass with time as your body adjusts to the new medication. If the symptoms persist, call your doctor.

ON THE HORIZON. Researchers are always looking for new and improved glucose-lowering pills. Currently, they are studying medications that block the body's absorption of fats. This can improve blood glucose control and help with weight loss and maintenance. Researchers are also investigating drugs to help the body's insulin work better and medications that increase the body's sensitivity to insulin. Stay informed on the latest developments by talking to your team and by looking for updates in diabetes magazines.

Insulin

Sometimes blood glucose levels are not controlled adequately with food planning, exercise, and glucose-lowering pills. When this happens, type II diabetes can be treated with a combination of glucose-lowering pills and insulin, or with insulin alone. You and your health care provider will decide which therapy you need based on your current level of control and your treatment goals. However, following a food plan and staying active are still a part of treatment when you are taking insulin. Taking insulin by injection does not mean you have type I diabetes. You are simply treating your type II diabetes with insulin.

It may seem odd that insulin injections would be helpful. After all, your pancreas still makes insulin, and your body may not be using the insulin effectively anyway. Why would adding more insulin help?

Think of it like this: Over time your pancreas makes less insulin than it used to, even though some insulin is still being made. Also, your body may be resistant to the insulin it makes. This is probable if you are overweight. Taking an insulin injection adds to your own dwindling insulin supply and helps overcome insulin resistance. The presence of more insulin also lowers blood glucose by signaling the liver to decrease the amount of glucose it produces.

WHAT IT MEANS FOR YOU. It's natural to feel a little afraid if you need to start taking insulin. Some people worry that the shots will hurt. Others wonder how they will fit insulin injections into their lives. Still others feel guilty if they haven't been taking good care of their diabetes. They think that is why they have to take insulin.

Most people find they adjust to taking insulin quite well once they work through their feelings. Taking insulin injections becomes a regular part of your daily routine. Insulin shots are rarely painful because the needles are very short and thin. You can barely feel it. Also, insulin shots are given into fatty tissue and not into muscle or a vein, as many people fear. Don't hesitate to ask questions and discuss your feelings about insulin with your diabetes care team. They can be a great source of support and encouragement to you, as can your family and friends.

When you start taking insulin, you will need to make some adjustments in your life. You might have to get up a few minutes earlier in the morning, and you'll need to remember to eat your meals on time. As you adjust to taking insulin, many of your concerns will fade, because you will probably feel better than ever. If insulin is able to help keep your blood glucose levels in your target range, you will have more energy and have a better sense of overall well-being. You will discover that the benefits of insulin therapy far outweigh any inconvenience you may feel.

ABOUT INJECTED INSULIN. We know that insulin is made in our pancreas, but what about the insulin that is injected? Where does that come from?

In the past, all insulin used for injections came from cow and pig pancreases. These animal insulins are only slightly different in structure from the insulin made by our bodies, and they work quite well. Today, most insulin used for injections is made in the laboratory. Advanced technology is used to "program" bacteria or yeast to make a very purified "human" insulin. The end result is an insulin that is identical in structure to what our bodies produce.

Though animal insulins are still available, it is usually recommended that you use human insulin. People are less likely to have allergic reactions or to develop antibodies to human insulin. Human insulin is always recommended for pregnant women and at times when insulin is going to be used in a temporary setting.

DOSES AND SCHEDULES. There is no one insulin therapy that works for everyone. Insulin doses and schedules for taking insulin are specifically designed for each individual. Your diabetes care team will work with you to determine how much insulin you need to take. Usually, insulin is started at low doses and is adjusted according to blood glucose testing results. It sometimes takes several weeks of adjustments to get the dose you need.

Some people temporarily feel worse or complain of blurry vision when they start taking insulin. This happens because their bodies are trying to get used to blood glucose levels that are lower and closer to normal, which is brought about by taking insulin. If you begin taking insulin, you may need patience to get through the first few weeks. But after a time of adjustment, most people feel better than they can remember feeling in a long time.

Different insulins have different action times. That is, each type of insulin begins to work at a certain time, peaks in effectiveness at a certain time, and leaves the body after a certain amount of time. Table 7.2 shows the different types of insulin and the action times of each.

Though some people may only take one insulin injection each day, most people need at least two injections per day to control their blood glucose. The two-shots-a-day insulin regimen offers more flexibility with eating and activity than one shot a day, and it usually gives better control. That's why more people use it. Usually, one shot is taken before breakfast and the other before the evening meal. Some people, however, take three or even four shots a day to get the control they need and want.

In most cases, each insulin shot is a combination of two insulins: short-acting and intermediate-acting. Both types of insulin can be drawn up together in one syringe. The short-acting insulin helps the body use the food that is about to be eaten. The intermediate-acting insulin helps keep a steady supply of insulin in the body between meals or overnight. Taken together, these insulins more closely imitate how a normal pancreas releases insulin during the day than the one-shot-a-day regimen does. For example, the graph in Figure 7.1 shows how regular and NPH insulins work in the two-shots-a-day regimen.

Insulin is also available in pre-mixed ratios of 70% NPH and 30% regular (called 70/30) and 50% NPH and 50% regular (called 50/50). Obviously this makes measuring insulin easier, but the pre-mixed combinations do not meet everyone's needs. Some

TABLE 7.2 **Types of Insulin**

Human Insulin	Begins to Work	Peak Effect	Duration of Effect
Very short acting (lispro)[1]	5–15 minutes	45–90 minutes	3–4 hours
Short acting (regular)	30–60 minutes	2–3 hours	4–6 hours
Intermediate acting (NPH or lente)	2–4 hours	4–12 hours	10–18 hours
Long acting (ultralente)	4–6 hours	small peak from 8–16 hours	up to 24 hours
Mixtures (70/30; 50/50)	30–60 minutes	2–12 hours	up to 18 hours

NOTE: This table summarizes the action time of various insulins. These times vary widely from person to person based on several factors, including the amount of insulin injected, site and depth of injection, skin temperature, and exercise.

[1] Lispro (Humalog®) is a new insulin that starts working very quickly once it is injected. It is expected to be available in 1996. Whereas it is recommended to take short-acting human insulin (regular) 30 minutes before eating, lispro is to be taken *at the meal*. This may make this type of insulin more convenient for some people.

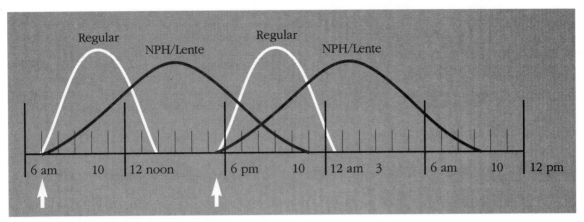

FIGURE 7.1 **Insulin Activity Graph**

people need to take more of one kind of insulin or less of another, and pre-mixed insulins do not allow for that flexibility.

LEARNING TO TAKE INSULIN. Insulin affects important aspects of your life—mainly when and how much you eat and exercise. You need special instruction to learn how to use insulin properly. You cannot just read the instructions on the bottle as you do for aspirin or other medications. Your diabetes care team will help you learn:

- what kind and amount of insulin to take;
- when to take your insulin;
- how to match your food with your insulin;
- how to prepare and take your insulin;
- where on your body to give yourself the injections;
- how to store your insulin;
- how to obtain the supplies you need to get started; and
- how to balance food, insulin, and activity.

Many people are concerned about hypoglycemia when they first start taking insulin. As with glucose-lowering pills, hypoglycemia does sometimes occur when you take insulin. The causes of hypoglycemia include taking too much insulin, not eating on schedule, or being more active than usual. Specifics on recognizing symptoms and treating hypoglycemia are on page 78. If you do start taking insulin, it is very important that you know how to recognize and treat hypoglycemia. If at all possible, teach the people you live and work with about hypoglycemia as well.

The sessions with your diabetes educator or dietitian are your time to learn all you need to know. During your visits, be sure to ask questions if anything seems unclear to you.

Taking insulin will help you manage your diabetes. It's like many of the other things we choose to do to live a healthier life—sometimes we resist healthy habits because they take too much time or seem like a nuisance. Taking insulin is one of those things that takes some getting used to. But the benefits of following your insulin schedule are worth the inconvenience. When you keep your diabetes under control, you will feel better and help to ensure your long-term health.

Key Points

- Treatment plans for people with type II diabetes include a food and activity plan and, sometimes, glucose-lowering pills or insulin injections.
- There are currently three kinds of glucose-lowering pills: Sulfonylureas, biguanides, and alpha glucosidase inhibitors.
- Glucose-lowering pills should not be used if you have type I diabetes, if you are pregnant or breast feeding, if you have kidney or liver disease or other serious medical problems, or if you drink excessive amounts of alcohol.
- The added insulin from injections lowers your blood glucose and helps overcome insulin resistance.
- The use of glucose-lowering pills or insulin injections may cause hypoglycemia, or low blood glucose.
- There are different types of insulin, each with a different action profile.
- Different insulins may be used in combination to get the best blood glucose control.

Part Three

WORKING TOWARD CONTROL

The Diabetes Control and Complications Trial (DCCT)

National Institutes of Health

The DCCT was the largest and most comprehensive diabetes study ever conducted. Spanning a decade, from 1983 to 1993, the study involved 1441 volunteers with type I diabetes (insulin-dependent diabetes mellitus) and 29 medical centers in the United States and Canada.

The study compared the effects of a standard therapy regimen and an intensive therapy regimen. Participants were randomly divided into these two groups. Those in the intensive therapy regimen achieved tight blood glucose control by:

- *testing their blood glucose four or more times a day;*
- *taking four daily insulin injections or used an insulin pump;*
- *adhering to a food/meal plan and exercise plan;*
- *adjusting their insulin doses according to their food intake and exercise; and*
- *visiting monthly with their diabetes care team.*

At the end of ten years, the study results showed that keeping blood glucose levels as close to normal as possible (intensive regimen) reduced eye disease by 76 percent, kidney disease by 50 percent, and nerve disease by 60 percent. In fact, it showed that any sustained lowering of blood glucose helps, even if the person has a history of poor control.

The DCCT's findings are hailed as significant proof that intensive blood glucose control will reduce or delay the onset of these diabetes complications. And researchers believe that people with type II diabetes will reap the same benefits from intensive blood glucose control.

Chapter 8

MONITORING YOUR BLOOD GLUCOSE

We use a variety of tools to check up on our health. A person who is trying to maintain or lose weight might use a bathroom scale regularly. Someone who is coming down with a cold or the flu might use a thermometer to check his or her temperature.

When you have diabetes, one of the most important tools you use to check on your health is self blood glucose monitoring (SBGM). SBGM is a simple blood test you do at home. It tells you what your blood glucose level is at the moment you test. Testing at regular times each day helps you keep track of your blood glucose levels throughout the day. It is the only way to know for sure what your levels are.

Recording the results of your blood glucose tests is also very important. Your blood glucose records can help you and your diabetes care team understand how food, activity, stress, and other factors affect your blood glucose levels. Your records also help you and your team decide when you may need to make changes in your treatment.

Testing your blood glucose level regularly and keeping a record of the results are two of the most important things you do to help manage your diabetes. When your blood glucose levels are within your target range, you feel better and have more energy than when they are not. You also lower your chances of developing the long-term health problems that diabetes can cause.

How to Test Your Blood Glucose

Self blood glucose monitoring begins with a single drop of blood. Blood is drawn from the finger using a lancing device. A lancing device is a small spring-loaded device with a tiny needle called a lancet.

Once the blood is drawn, you use one of two methods to test: Either a blood glucose meter or a visual test strip. Blood glucose meters are easy to use and give an exact reading of your blood glucose level. A drop of blood is placed on a test strip and the meter does the rest! Your blood glucose level is displayed on a digital readout.

Meters are available with a wide variety of features. Some have a built-in memory to save your test results. You or your diabetes care team can then download the data into a computer for analysis. Meters also come in a wide variety of sizes and price ranges.

Testing Tips

- *Do not clean the site with alcohol before drawing blood. Alcohol can change your test results and can dry out your skin. Washing with soap and water is all that is needed.*

- *Change the site each time you draw blood so that no one area becomes sore. The sides and ends of your fingertips are less sensitive than the center.*

- *Keep your test strips dry in a vial or foil wrapper until you are ready to do a test. Air and humidity can ruin the strip and give you inaccurate results.*

- *Do not leave your strips in extreme heat or cold, and be sure to use them before the expiration date printed on the package.*

- *Get an adequate drop of blood. Your results can be inaccurate if you do not apply enough blood to the test strip.*

- *Time the test according to the manufacturer's directions.*

- *Dispose of used lancets by placing them in an empty metal or hard plastic container. Plastic soda pop or milk bottles work well. Cap the container or tape it shut and label it "needles" before throwing it in the garbage. You also may buy containers made specifically for disposing of needles through medical supply companies.*

Your diabetes care team can help you choose the meter that is best for you.

Visual strips work by placing a drop of blood on the strip. Chemicals in the strip interact with the blood to change the color of the paper. You then match the color on the strip to the color bars on the test strip bottle to find your approximate blood glucose level.

Visual strips don't give you a specific blood glucose number, such as 138 mg/dl, the way meters do. Instead, they give you a blood glucose range, such as 120 to 180 mg/dl (6.7 to 10 mM/L). Visual testing may be all you need if your diabetes is under good control, or if you don't need an exact reading of your blood glucose level.

Accurate test results depend on good testing technique. Your diabetes care team will teach you how to use your specific meter or visual test strips. Even if you've been testing for a long time, you should have someone from your diabetes care team watch you do it at each visit to make sure you continue to use the proper technique.

> **Steps for Self-Testing**
>
> **Step 1** *Wash the test site with soap and water. Warm water helps increase blood flow to the area.*
>
> **Step 2** *Puncture the skin with the lancing device.*
>
> **Step 3** *Gently massage the area until a large drop of blood forms.*
>
> **Step 4** *Place the drop on the test strip.*
>
> **Step 5** *Follow the manufacturer's instructions for timing the test and taking the reading.*
>
> **Step 6** *Record the results in your record book.*

Keeping Good Records

Self blood glucose monitoring is most helpful when you keep a record of the results. By writing down your results each time you test, you will have an accurate picture of your day-to-day blood glucose levels. But good record keeping is more than just writing down numbers. Your blood glucose test results provide important information that helps guide your day-to-day management decisions.

Most record books have columns for recording your test time and results; your diabetes medication and dose, if any; and any information about food or activity that might be important. Your diabetes care team will probably recommend or provide you with a record book for keeping track of your results. Many meters also come with record books. A sample record book is shown in Figure 8.1.

Seeing your blood glucose levels written down in black and white can be very powerful. It can show you at a glance when your blood glucose level is in your target range and when it is not. This can have both positive and negative effects. On the plus side, you are aware of times when you may need to make adjustments in your lifestyle choices or your treatment plan to improve your diabetes control. On the down side, you may become overly concerned or have feelings of failure whenever your blood glucose level is higher or lower than you'd like. If you feel this way, you may be tempted to test only when you are sure you're going to be happy with the result. You may even be tempted to write down false numbers—all in your target range.

Month Date	A.M. Medication	A.M. BG Before	A.M. BG After	Notes	Midday Medication	Midday BG Before	Midday BG After	Notes
6/10	Glyburide 10 mg	7:00 130						
6/13		8:15 120						late lunch
6/16		7:45 135						walk 45 min
6/19		7:00 122	10:00 shaky — skipped breakfast BG 68					
6/22		7:00 114						

FIGURE 8.1 **Record Book Sample (page one). Blood glucose levels are recorded in mg/dl.**

But having a record book filled with all "perfect scores" isn't the point of SBGM or record keeping. Blood glucose test results should not be considered "good" or "bad," and your record book is not a report card. What you need is a record book filled with readings that show your real day-to-day blood glucose levels. Without accurate records, you and your diabetes care team won't know when your treatment plan is working and when it's not.

When to Test

Your blood glucose levels can vary widely throughout the day. Each test is just a snapshot of your blood glucose level at that moment, so testing once a day usually is not enough. To get the

P.M. Medication	P.M. BG		Notes	Evening Medication	Snack BG		Notes
	Before	After			Before	After	
	5:00	7:00					
Glyburide 5 mg	87	195	out to dinner				walked at mall
	5:30	7:30					
	145	179					
	5:00	7:00					
	61	150	felt shaky				
	5:00	6:45					
	106	160					
	5:15	7:15					
	98	167					walk after supper 35 min

FIGURE 8.1 **Record Book Sample (page two)**

whole picture of your blood glucose control and how your levels are affected by what you eat and do, you need to test more often.

The goals of testing are to have the data you need to evaluate the effectiveness of your treatment and to help you reach your target blood glucose goals. Work with your diabetes care team to develop a testing schedule that meets your needs. Common testing times include:

- first thing in the morning;
- before meals; and/or
- one to two hours after meals.

If you take insulin, it is recommended that you test four times a day. An example of this would be testing before each meal and before your evening snack. If you do not take insulin, you may test less often. For example, test before breakfast, before your main meal, and one to two hours after finishing your main meal (for a total of three blood tests a day).

Special Times to Test

Sometimes you need to test at times beyond your regular routine. These are times when your blood glucose levels might be higher or lower than usual because of unusual activities or circumstances. Pay special attention to your blood glucose levels at these times.

WHEN YOU FEEL SYMPTOMS OF HYPOGLYCEMIA (LOW BLOOD GLUCOSE). Sometimes people think they are having a hypoglycemic reaction when they are not. Excitement, stress, and some medications may cause feelings similar to hypoglycemic symptoms. Before treating for hypoglycemia, you should always test your blood glucose level to be sure your symptoms really are caused by a low blood glucose level and not by something else. If you feel symptoms of hypoglycemia and your blood glucose level is below 80 mg/dl (4.4 mM/L), you need to treat it. *Any time* your blood glucose level is below 70 mg/dl (3.9 mM/L), it should be treated, whether you have symptoms or not. If you can't test and you feel that you're low, you should treat the symptoms. Guidelines for treating hypoglycemia are on page 78.

WHEN YOU ARE SICK. Even a simple cold can cause problems with your blood glucose control. Whenever you feel under the weather, test your blood glucose level three to five times throughout the day to be sure it isn't getting too high. Blood glucose levels often are higher when you are sick. If you do develop hyperglycemia (high blood glucose), you may need to test even more often as you treat the problem. You should call your diabetes care team any time your blood glucose level is over 240 mg/dl (13.3 mM/L) when you are sick.

WHEN YOUR SCHEDULE CHANGES. Times of stress or changes in your daily routine can affect your blood glucose control. Check with your diabetes care team whenever you make major changes in your daily routine. They can give you advice on how to adjust your treatment plan to best meet the needs caused by the change. Some things that may signal the need to test more often or at different times are when you are:

- changing the dose or timing of diabetes medications;
- changing your physical activity;
- starting a new job;
- working a new shift;
- traveling through different time zones; or
- experiencing any unusual stress in your family due to a death, illness, or divorce, etc.

WHEN YOU ARE ON VACATION. You can take a vacation from work, home, the family, or just your daily routine. But vacations are the worst times to take a break from SBGM. Changes in your daily routine, the foods you eat, and your level of activity while you are on vacation make testing your blood glucose all the more important. Some people even find that this is true for weekends and work holidays. Whenever your schedule is different from your usual routine, you need to be sure to monitor your blood glucose accordingly.

Getting the Most from Monitoring

The payoff for testing your blood glucose and keeping good records is knowing how well your treatment plan is working each day. In order to do this, you need to know what you are aiming for.

TABLE 8.1 **Target Blood Glucose Ranges**

Time of Day	Suggested Target	My Target
Fasting and before meals	80-140 mg/dl (4.4-7.8 mM/L)	
1-2 hours after meals	100-180 mg/dl (5.5-10 mM/L)	

We introduced target blood glucose ranges in Chapter 2 and have discussed them throughout the book. You need to be sure you know what your target blood glucose ranges are. Talk with your health care provider to set your targets, then record them in the space provided in Table 8.1. The suggested ranges are shown as a guideline.

But what do you do when your blood glucose level is outside your target range? First, record it accurately. Also write down in your record book anything you can think of that might explain the reading. Table 8.2 shows some of the things that can cause higher or lower blood glucose levels. You also may notice other things particular to you and to your lifestyle that affect your blood glucose levels. Experiment by testing at different times of the day and after eating different types of foods to see how your blood glucose level is affected.

It is not uncommon to have a few readings outside your target range. The key is to examine each occurrence, whether it is a high or low blood glucose level, and to try to understand it and learn

TABLE 8.2 **Blood Glucose Levels**

Blood Glucose Levels May Be Higher When:	Blood Glucose Levels May Be Lower When:
• you eat more food than usual; • you exercise less than usual; • you are under emotional or physical stress; • you take too little glucose-lowering medication or insulin; or • you are ill.	• you eat less food than usual; • you exercise more than usual; • you delay or skip a meal or snack; or • you take too much glucose-lowering medication or insulin.

from it. This can help you make changes that may prevent the same thing from happening again. Your blood glucose records are very helpful for this. They can help you identify patterns of high or low blood glucose levels and pinpoint what is working for you and what is not.

One way to analyze your blood glucose readings is to look at one week in your record book and mark with a highlighter pen all the numbers that are within your target range. Then ask yourself these questions:

- Are more than half of all the numbers within my target range?
- Are the numbers that are not within my range generally higher or lower than my range?
- Can I explain high or low readings by identifying unusual eating or activity patterns—or was I ill?
- How do my readings at specific times of the day compare from day to day? For instance, how do all my morning readings compare?
- Is there a difference in my levels between weekdays and weekends?

The answers to these questions can help you determine what problem spots you have, if any. Then you can figure out what to do to correct any problems. For instance, you may notice that your blood glucose level is consistently high before dinner. In this case, you would look at your afternoon routine, including what, how much, and when you ate and how active you were. Then you would think about adjustments you might make to help bring your before-dinner readings into your target range. You could eat a smaller mid-afternoon snack or eat your snack earlier in the afternoon. Another option might be to take a brisk mid-afternoon walk.

If you notice high blood glucose levels, ask yourself these questions to help determine what might be causing them and what you might do about it:

- Am I following my food plan? Does it make a difference in my readings when I follow my food plan versus when I do not?
- Is there a change I could make in the timing of my meals or snacks or in the amount of food I eat that might improve my readings? Am I willing to make the change?

• Is there a change I could make in the timing or amount of my activity that might improve my readings? Am I willing to make the change?

• Is there anything else going on that might make my readings go up, such as an illness (flu, cold, infection) or stress?

To lower blood glucose levels:

• *Be more active overall and add more planned activity to your daily routine.*

• *Spread carbohydrate foods more evenly throughout the day or eat less carbohydrate if necessary.*

• *Take your diabetes medications, if any, at the prescribed times.*

It is sometimes hard to solve the puzzle of high blood glucose readings. If you are not sure why your levels are high, or if you are doing all you can and your numbers remain high, discuss the situation with your diabetes care team. You may need to make a change in your treatment plan, such as adding or adjusting a diabetes medication. Even if you feel fine, always call your physician if *most* of your blood glucose readings are above 240 mg/dl (13.3 mM/L) for three days in a row.

You may also see a pattern of low blood glucose readings in your record book. If you take glucose-lowering pills or insulin and you are getting blood glucose readings that are too low (below 70 mg/dl or 3.9 mM/L, or below your target range), ask yourself these questions:

• Am I following my food plan?
• Have I delayed or skipped meals or snacks?
• Have I lost weight?
• Am I taking my diabetes medication as prescribed?
• Do I need a change in my diabetes medication timing or dose?

SBGM and your blood glucose records put you in charge of your diabetes. Learn to understand and use the numbers to help keep your diabetes in the best control you can.

Handling Hypoglycemia

You do not need to worry about low blood glucose levels if you are treating your diabetes with a food plan and exercise alone. However, if you take glucose-lowering pills or inject insulin, it is possible for your blood glucose level to get too low. The causes of low blood glucose are listed in Table 8.2 on page 76.

You need to treat for hypoglycemia whenever your blood glucose level is below 70 mg/dl (3.9 mM/L). If you have symptoms of hypoglycemia and your blood glucose is either below 80 mg/dl (4.4 mM/L) or below your target range, you also should treat for hypoglycemia. Early symptoms of hypoglycemia are:

- paleness;
- feeling shaky and weak;
- sweating;
- dizziness;
- fast heartbeat;
- hunger; and
- tingling or numb lips.

Having some or all of these symptoms means that your brain and nervous system are not getting enough glucose. If untreated, you might have a hard time walking or speaking. You may get confused.

Know the symptoms of hypoglycemia and be prepared to treat them. If you feel any of the symptoms, test your blood. Any time your blood glucose level is below 70 mg/dl (3.9 mM/L), eat or drink something that contains 15 grams of carbohydrate. Liquid or soft foods are the best choices.

It's easy to overtreat low blood glucose. You may be feeling anxious and your body may be telling you to eat. However, if you eat too much, your blood glucose levels can get too high. The best thing to do when you feel symptoms of low blood glucose is to eat the suggested serving of food and wait quietly for it to take effect. This takes about ten to fifteen minutes. Then test your blood again.

If your second test is above 70 mg/dl (3.9 mM/L) and you feel better, you can go about what you were doing. If your test is still below 70 mg/dl, eat another carbohydrate food. After fifteen minutes, test again. If you still have low blood glucose after three tests, call your doctor.

Check with your diabetes care team if you have frequent or severe hypoglycemia. You may need to make some changes in your treatment plan.

Foods and Beverages for Treating Hypoglycemia

- *3 glucose tablets*
- *1/2 cup of fruit juice*
- *1/2 cup regular soft drink (not diet)*
- *1 cup skim milk*
- *6 to 7 hard candies*
- *6 small sugar cubes*
- *8 to 10 jelly beans*
- *1 tablespoon of honey*
- *1 small tube of cake frosting*

PREVENTION. Controlling your diabetes requires a delicate balance of food, exercise, and insulin (natural or injected). Together, you and your diabetes care team have developed a treatment plan designed to help you keep that balance. The best thing you can do to prevent hypoglycemia is to follow your plan.

Be alert to changes in your schedule. If you're called into a meeting when it's time for your snack, take it with you. Or if you end up in a volleyball match at a family picnic or out in the garden too long, eat something extra. It may sometimes feel like an imposition or just too much trouble, but small adjustments like these can help you avoid hypoglycemia. Be prepared. Carry a carbohydrate food with you at all times. Hard candies or glucose tablets are easy to carry in a pocket, briefcase, or purse.

Hypoglycemia Prevention Guidelines

- *Test your blood glucose level routinely.*
- *Follow your prescribed food plan.*
- *Do not delay meals or snacks.*
- *If you take insulin, measure it carefully and take the correct amounts.*
- *Take other medications exactly as prescribed.*
- *Plan for exercise.*
- *Eat food when you drink wine, beer, or liquor.*
- *Test your blood glucose level before driving.*

DRIVING PRECAUTIONS. Reactions are especially hazardous while driving. It is important to take precautions. If you can, test your blood glucose level before you drive. Eat a small snack if your glucose level is below 80 mg/dl (4.4 mM/L). If you can't test and it's been more than two hours since your last meal or snack, eat a snack anyway, just in case. When driving long distances, eat a small snack every two to three hours.

To be safe, always keep some food in your car. Hard candies, a small box of raisins, or glucose tablets should have a permanent home in your glove compartment.

Many states have established laws related to diabetes and driving. These laws vary from state to state. For information on the driving laws in your state, call your Department of Public Safety.

Maintaining Your Meter

In order to get an accurate picture of your blood glucose control, you need to be sure the readings you are getting from your meter truly reflect actual values. You can do this by following a few simple guidelines for meter maintenance.

1. *Clean your meter.* It's recommended that you do this at least once a week. Follow the meter's instructions for cleaning.

2. *Check your meter function.* Some meters have two ways to check that the meter system is working. One way is to use a check strip to make sure the meter is operating properly. Check your meter instruction book for the specific directions. The other way is to check your meter and test strips using glucose control solutions. This is done to assure the meter and strips are working together properly. The control solution is a liquid that has a pre-determined amount of glucose in it. When you use this solution on the test strip, you are checking to see if the machine reads the "glucose" within the expected range. (The expected ranges are usually listed on your vial of strips.) When the reading is within the expected range, you can be confident in the accuracy of your meter readings.

   Check with the control solution when:
   • you open a new vial of strips;
   • you forget to replace the cap on the strip vial and the bottle has been left open for more than a few minutes;
   • you question the accuracy of the results you are getting; or
   • you drop the meter.

3. *Once a year, compare a test you do on your meter against a laboratory blood glucose test.* The comparison will show if you are getting accurate results from your testing method. To do this, take your blood testing supplies with you when you are having a blood test as part of a visit to your diabetes care team. Do your finger stick test within five minutes of the time blood is drawn from your arm for a laboratory blood test. To get an accurate comparison, the tests should be done at a time when you have not had food or beverages for at least ten to twelve hours before the blood test. When you get the results of both tests, you can compare them to see whether your self test result is in line with the lab test result. It is common for there to be a slight difference, but the two should not be too far off. If you see more than a twenty percent difference, talk to your health care provider.

Hemoglobin A$_{1c}$ Test

In addition to testing your blood glucose yourself, it is important to have a glycosylated hemoglobin test (hemoglobin A$_{1c}$) every three to four months. This test is done in a laboratory and shows your average blood glucose level over the past six to ten weeks. Your hemoglobin A$_{1c}$ results help you and your diabetes care team know if your treatment plan is working. You can read more about this test in Chapter 14 or you can obtain information from your health care provider.

Key Points

- Self blood glucose monitoring (SBGM) is a blood test you do at home that tells you what your blood glucose level is at the moment you test.
- There are two methods used to test: A blood glucose meter or a visual test strip.
- It is important to keep careful records of your blood glucose readings so that you and your diabetes care team can tell if your treatment plan is working or not.
- Your diabetes care team can help you decide when and how often you need to test.
- In addition to your regular testing schedule, you need to test more often when you feel symptoms of hypoglycemia, when you're sick, when your schedule changes, and when you're on vacation.
- When you have readings outside of your target range, try to figure out what might have caused them.
- Treat yourself for hypoglycemia whenever your blood glucose level is below 70 mg/dl (3.9 mM/L). If you have symptoms of hypoglycemia and your blood glucose is either below 80 mg/dl (4.4 mM/L) or below your target range, you also should treat for hypoglycemia.

Chapter 9

DEVELOPING YOUR FOOD PLAN

In Chapter 4 you learned about the nutrients in food and how what you eat affects your blood glucose and health. Now let's use that knowledge to work on developing your food plan.

Your food plan combines the goals of nutrition in diabetes with methods to reach those goals. It is not a set menu or a diet. Rather, it is a guide for choosing foods and serving sizes wisely. It suggests how many servings from different food groups to eat for meals and snacks so that you meet your nutrition needs and maintain blood glucose control.

Your food plan is designed according to your lifestyle, food preferences, and health goals. It is a reasonable compromise between what, when, and how much food you usually eat, and what, when, and how much food will help you reach your

TABLE 9.1 **Nutrition Goals**

Goals of Nutrition in Diabetes	How to Achieve Nutrition Goals
• To keep blood glucose levels as close to normal as possible • To achieve healthy blood fat levels • To help you get to and stay at a reasonable weight • To meet nutrition needs	• Space food intake throughout the day • Eat smaller amounts of food at a time • Eat less food overall • Eat less saturated fat • Choose a variety of foods • Eat a consistent amount of carbohydrate at meals and snacks • Get and stay physically active

diabetes management goals. The key to maintaining blood glucose control is to eat consistently throughout the day and from day-to-day. But that doesn't mean what you eat has to be boring.

Carbohydrate Counting

We've said it many times, but it's worth saying again: Carbohydrate affects blood glucose levels more than other food nutrients. Too much carbohydrate at any one time can overload your insulin supply and cause high blood glucose levels. Likewise, too little carbohydrate can cause your blood glucose level to go too low and make you feel hungry.

Your food plan includes guidelines for how many carbohydrate choices to eat and when to eat them. A *carbohydrate choice* is a serving of food (starch, fruit, or milk) that contains 15 grams of carbohydrate. (See Table 9.3 on page 88 for specific carbohydrate foods and servings sizes.) Eating about the same amount of carbohydrate for your daily meals and snacks can help you control your blood glucose levels. A healthful food plan generally includes three to four carbohydrate choices per meal and one to two carbohydrate choices at planned snack times.

Your food plan will help you learn to count the carbohydrate choices you eat. By counting carbohydrate choices and testing your blood glucose levels, you will know how well your body is using carbohydrate for energy. With experience, you will learn how to make adjustments in your food choices, activity, or even medications for the best blood glucose control. For instance, if your blood glucose is high after eating a large serving of pasta or potatoes, you might eat less carbohydrate the next time, or take a brisk walk after eating to help lower your blood glucose level.

One of the greatest things about carbohydrate counting is that you have a lot of flexibility in the food choices you make. Eating a variety of foods is very important for good nutrition and good health, and with carbohydrate counting you can get that variety. For example, you can eat six cups of popped corn as a snack, if that's what you want. You just have to count the carbohydrate in the popped corn (two carbohydrate choices) and include it as part of your food plan for that day. The next day, you may decide to have a small cookie and a glass of milk (two carbohydrate

TABLE 9.2 **Carbohydrate Choices**

2 Carbohydrate Choices	3 Carbohydrate Choices	4 Carbohydrate Choices
6 cups plain popped corn (2 servings of 3 cups each) [2]	1 cup broth based soup [1]; 6 saltine crackers [1]; and 1 apple [1]	2 pieces of toast [2]; 1/2 cup orange juice [1]; and 1 cup milk [1]
OR	OR	OR
1 small cookie [1] and 1 cup milk [1]	1 1/2 cups cooked pasta (3 servings of 1/2 cup each) [3]	2 six-inch tortillas (2 servings of 1 tortilla each) [2] and 1 cup cooked pinto beans (2 servings of 1/2 cup each) [2]

choices) for your snack. That would be okay because it has the same amount of carbohydrate as the six cups of popped corn.

Knowing what a carbohydrate choice is includes knowing what foods have carbohydrate in them and how much of each food is one carbohydrate choice. Portions are very important. Table 9.2 shows examples of what makes up two, three, or four carbohydrate choices. The number in brackets shows how many carbohydrate choices each item is.

Your Food Plan

Now you are ready to work on your food plan. Because your food plan is based on your personal eating habits and patterns, we will start by looking at how you currently eat. (If you haven't already done so, it is a good idea to meet with a registered dietitian and work on your food plan together. She or he can assist you in determining what, when, and how much to eat.[1])

Use the Food Plan Worksheet on page 86 to write an example of the food you eat and drink in a typical day. Think carefully and write down everything that you eat. Also, estimate the amount you

---

[1] To find a registered dietitian in your area, call the American Dietetic Association at 1-800-366-1655 or your local American Diabetes Association. In Canada, call your local Canadian Diabetes Association branch or hospital.

Food Plan Worksheet

My Typical Breakfast

Food/Amount	Starch	Fruit	Milk	Vegetable	Meat	Fat
_____	_____	_____	_____	_____	_____	_____
_____	_____	_____	_____	_____	_____	_____
_____	_____	_____	_____	_____	_____	_____

Total carbohydrate choices (starch, fruit, and milk): _____

My Typical Mid-Morning Snack

Food/Amount	Starch	Fruit	Milk	Vegetable	Meat	Fat
_____	_____	_____	_____	_____	_____	_____

Total carbohydrate choices (starch, fruit, and milk): _____

My Typical Midday Meal

Food/Amount	Starch	Fruit	Milk	Vegetable	Meat	Fat
_____	_____	_____	_____	_____	_____	_____
_____	_____	_____	_____	_____	_____	_____
_____	_____	_____	_____	_____	_____	_____

Total carbohydrate choices (starch, fruit, and milk): _____

My Typical Mid-Afternoon Snack

Food/Amount	Starch	Fruit	Milk	Vegetable	Meat	Fat
_____	_____	_____	_____	_____	_____	_____

Total carbohydrate choices (starch, fruit, and milk): _____

My Typical Evening Meal

Food/Amount	Starch	Fruit	Milk	Vegetable	Meat	Fat
_____	_____	_____	_____	_____	_____	_____
_____	_____	_____	_____	_____	_____	_____
_____	_____	_____	_____	_____	_____	_____

Total carbohydrate choices (starch, fruit, and milk): _____

My Typical Evening Snack

Food/Amount	Starch	Fruit	Milk	Vegetable	Meat	Fat
_____	_____	_____	_____	_____	_____	_____

Total carbohydrate choices (starch, fruit, and milk): _____

	Starch	Fruit	Milk	Vegetable	Meat	Fat
DAILY TOTALS	_____	_____	_____	_____	_____	_____

eat (one-half banana, one whole banana, one cup milk, etc.) and write that down, too. For instance, a sandwich may include two pieces of bread, two ounces of turkey, one ounce of cheese, two teaspoons of mayonnaise, and lettuce.

Now you are ready to evaluate your typical day's food intake to determine what, when, and how much you currently eat. To do this, we will look at carbohydrate choices, daily calories, and the quality of nutrition.

STEP 1: CARBOHYDRATE CHOICES Circle the foods listed on your worksheet that contain carbohydrate. Write how many carbohydrate choices each circled item is in the appropriate column: starch, fruit, or milk. (Table 9.3 identifies the different foods and gives serving sizes that equal one carbohydrate choice.) Add up the carbohydrate choices for each meal and each snack and write the total in the space provided on the worksheet.

Are your carbohydrate choices similar to these guidelines? (circle one)

Three to four carbohydrate choices for each meal?   yes   no
One to two carbohydrate choices for each snack?   yes   no

STEP 2: DAILY CALORIES Look at the rest of the foods listed on your worksheet. Count the servings of vegetables, meat, and fat you eat for each meal and each snack. Table 9.3 will help with serving sizes. Write the number of servings in the appropriate columns on the worksheet.

Add up the total servings of each type of food (starch, fruit, milk, vegetable, meat, fat) that you eat in a day and write the numbers in the spaces at the bottom of the worksheet. For example, add down the starch column to get the total starch servings for all the meals and snacks on your worksheet. Put the daily totals in the Calorie Calculator on page 91 and multiply to find the number of calories provided by each type of food. Then add up the total daily calories and write the number in the Calorie Calculator.

The amount of calories you need is determined by your weight, age, gender, and activity level. Most people need about ten to fifteen calories per pound of body weight. Now compare your total daily calories in the Calorie Counter to the calorie range listed for your weight in Table 9.4 (page 91).

TABLE 9.3 **Food Choices**

CARBOHYDRATE CHOICES

Starch Group
(6 or more servings a day)
1 serving = 15 grams carbohydrate, variable protein, 60-90 calories

Bagel or English muffin	1 half or 1 oz.
Bread, slice or roll	1 or 1 oz.
Cereal, cooked	1/2 cup
Cereal, unsweetened, ready-to-eat	3/4 cup
Corn, cooked	1/2 cup
Crackers, snack ♠	4-5
Dried beans, cooked	1/2 cup (also 1 meat)
Graham crackers	3 squares
Hamburger or hot dog bun	1 half or 1 oz.
Muffin, small ♠	1 (1 1/2 oz.)
Pancakes (4" across) ♠	2
Pasta, cooked (macaroni, noodles, spaghetti)	1/2 cup
Peas, green, cooked	1/2 cup
Popcorn, unbuttered	3 cups
Potato, small	1 (3 oz.)
Potato, mashed	1/2 cup
Rice, cooked	1/3 cup
Squash, winter, cooked	1 cup
Taco shells, 6" across ♠	2
Tortilla (6" across)	1
Waffles (4 1/2" across) ♠	1

Fruit Group (2-4 servings a day)
1 serving = 15 grams carbohydrate, 60-90 calories

Banana	1/2 medium
Berries or melon	1 cup
Canned fruit in juice or water	1/2 cup
Dried fruit	1/4 cup
Fresh fruit	1 medium
Fruit juice	1/3 to 1/2 cup
Grapes or cherries	12 to 15
Raisins	2 Tbsp.

Milk Group (2-3 servings a day)
1 serving = 12-15 grams carbohydrate, 8 grams protein, 60-90 calories

Milk, skim or low-fat	1 cup (8 oz.)
Yogurt, low-fat, artificially sweetened	3/4 to 1 cup (6-8 oz.)
Yogurt, plain, low-fat	3/4 to 1 cup (6-8 oz.)

More Carbohydrate Choices
1 serving = 15 grams carbohydrate. Protein, fat, and calories will vary.

Cake, no icing, 2" square ♠	1 piece
Casserole or hot dish ♠	1/2 cup (also 1 meat)
Chili	1/2 cup (also 1 meat)
Cookie, 3" across ♠	1
Frozen yogurt, low-fat or fat-free	1/3 cup
Ice cream or light ice cream ♠	1/2 cup
Maple syrup, honey, or table sugar	1 Tbsp.
Pizza, thin crust, medium ♠	1 slice or 1/8 pizza (also 1 meat)
Soup, broth-based ▼	1 cup
Soup, milk-based ♠ ▼	1 cup
Soup, bean-based ▼	1 cup (also 1 meat)
Spaghetti or pasta sauce, canned ♠ ▼	1/2 cup

TABLE 9.3 **Food Choices (cont'd.)**

OTHER FOOD CHOICES

Vegetables (3-5 servings a day)

1 serving = 5 grams carbohydrate, 2 grams protein, 25 calories. (One serving is 1/2 cup cooked or 1 cup raw. You may choose one vegetable or an assortment. Unless you eat more than three servings at one meal or snack, they are "free.")

Asparagus	Mushrooms
Beets	Onions
Broccoli	Pea pods
Cabbage	Peppers
Carrots	Radishes
Cauliflower	Salad greens
Celery	(lettuce, spinach)
Cucumbers	Tomatoes
Green beans	Turnips
Greens (collard, kale,	Zucchini
mustard, spinach, turnip)	

Fats (Limit to 3-5 servings a day)

1 serving = 5 grams fat, 45 calories

Butter*	1 tsp.
Cream cheese*	1 Tbsp.
Cream, table or light*	2 Tbsp.
Gravy*	2 Tbsp.
Margarine	1 tsp.
Margarine, low-fat	1 Tbsp.
Mayonnaise	1 tsp.
Mayonnaise, reduced-fat	1 Tbsp.
Nuts	1 Tbsp.
Oil	1 tsp.
Peanut butter	2 tsp.
Salad dressing	1 Tbsp.
Salad dressing, reduced-fat	2 Tbsp.
Sour cream*	2 Tbsp.
Sunflower seeds	1 Tbsp.

*Saturated fats

Meat/Meat Substitutes (up to 6 ounces a day)

1 ounce = 7 grams protein, 3-8 grams fat, 50-100 calories

MEATS

Beef	Pork
Fish	Poultry (no skin)
Ham ▼	Seafood
Lamb	Veal

MEAT SUBSTITUTES

Each item equals 1 oz. meat

Cottage cheese	1/4 cup
Reduced fat/part skim cheeses	1 oz.
Egg	1
Peanut butter ♠	2 Tbsp.
Tuna, salmon (water packed)	1/4 cup (1 oz.)

Meats should be baked, broiled, roasted or grilled. One serving of 3 ounces is:
- about the size of a deck of cards
- 1 medium pork chop
- 1 leg and 1 thigh or 1/2 of a whole breast of chicken
- 1/4 pound (weight before cooking) ground meat
- 1 medium unbreaded fish fillet

♠ also has 1 fat
▼ high sodium

TABLE 9.3 **Food Choices (cont'd.)**

FREE FOODS

Free foods are foods or beverages with fewer than 20 calories or fewer than 5 grams carbohydrate per serving. They have little or no effect on blood glucose levels.

Unlimited

Beverages	*Seasonings*	*Sweet Substitutes*
Bouillon ▼	Butter-flavored sprinkles	Gelatin desserts, sugar-free
Broth ▼	Butter-flavored sprays	Gum, sugar-free
Club soda	Flavoring extracts	Popsicles, sugar-free
Coffee	Herbs and spices	Sugar substitutes
Drink mixes, sugar-free	Mustard, prepared	
Mineral water	Nonstick cooking spray	
Soft drinks, diet	Soy sauce ▼	
Tea	Vinegar	
Tonic water, sugar-free	Wine, used in cooking	

Limit to 2-3 Times a Day

Fat-free Foods

Cream cheese, fat-free	1 Tbsp.
Creamers, non-dairy	1 Tbsp.
Mayonnaise, fat-free	1 Tbsp.
Salad dressing, fat-free	1 Tbsp.
Salsa	1/4 cup
Sour cream, fat-free	1 Tbsp.

Sweet Substitutes

Cocoa powder	1 Tbsp.
Jam or jelly, low sugar or light	1 to 2 tsp.
Syrup, sugar-free	2 Tbsp.
Whipped topping	1 Tbsp.
Yogurt, plain	2 Tbsp.

Condiments

Catsup	1 Tbsp.
Dill pickle ▼	1 large
Taco sauce	1 Tbsp.

♠ also has 1 fat
▼ high sodium

Calorie Calculator					
Food	Servings	X	Calories/Serving	=	Calories
Starch		X	80	=	
Fruit		X	60	=	
Milk		X	90	=	
Vegetable		X	25	=	
Meat		X	75	=	
Fat		X	45	=	
		Total Daily Calories		=	_____

TABLE 9.4 **Daily Calorie Needs**

Weight	Calorie Range
125	1600-1900
150	1900-2300
175	2100-2600
200	2200-2600
225	2250-2700
250	2500-2700
275	2500-3000
300	3000-3600
325	3250-3900
350	3500-4200

Daily calorie needs represent the number of calories you need each day to maintain your current weight. If you want to lose weight, you may cut your daily calories by 250 to 500. This will result in a weight loss of one-half to one pound per week. Increasing your aerobic activity will also help with weight loss.

STEP 3: NUTRITION Carbohydrates are important for maintaining a healthful diet and good blood glucose control, yet they are only part of your total food plan. A healthful food plan also includes daily food choices from the vegetable, meat/meat substitutes, and fat (careful amounts) groups. The recommended daily servings of each are shown on the food pyramid.

Compare the daily total servings of the different types of foods on your worksheet to the number of servings recommended in the food pyramid. (circle one)

Are you eating six or more servings from the grains/beans/starchy vegetables (starch) group each day?   yes   no

Are you eating two to four fruit servings each day?   yes   no

Are you eating two to three milk servings each day?   yes   no

Are you eating three to five vegetable servings each day?   yes   no

Are you eating six or fewer ounces of meat each day?   yes   no

Are you eating five or fewer fat servings each day?   yes   no

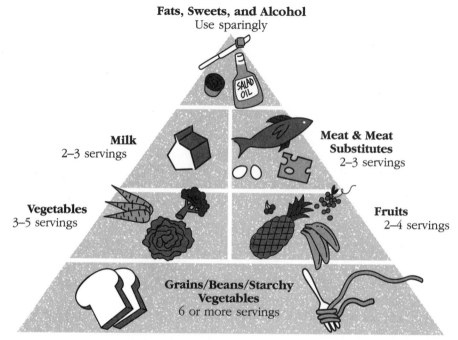

FIGURE 9.1 **Food Guide Pyramid**
Adapted from *Food Guide Pyramid,* © 1994, U.S. Department of Agriculture

PUTTING IT ALL TOGETHER. If you answered yes to the questions in Steps 1, 2, and 3, you have a good start on following a healthful food plan. Continue to follow that pattern of eating.

If you are not able to answer yes to all of the questions, identify the area that you need to change. Then think of what you can do to improve in that area. For example, perhaps you don't eat many vegetables. You could try to add a vegetable to each midday meal. Or maybe you are eating too much meat because your serving sizes are too big. You could begin weighing or measuring your meat servings until you get used to the recommended serving sizes.

As an example of how a food plan can help you, read about Marty's eating habits and then look at his food plan.

Shortly after Marty was diagnosed as having type II diabetes, he met with a dietitian to learn about diabetes and to design a food plan. Marty and his dietitian determined that Marty's daily servings of carbohydrate, meat, and fat were within the guidelines given in the food pyramid. His total calories were also adequate for his needs. One problem they did discover was that Marty was in the habit of skipping breakfast. He also ate most of his food, and nearly all his carbohydrate foods, between his evening meal and bedtime.

The dietitian explained that Marty might be overloading his body's insulin supply by eating a lot of food within the short period of time between the evening meal and bedtime. It was further explained that Marty would have a better chance of hitting his blood glucose targets if he spread his food intake throughout the day. Marty agreed to change his habits by eating breakfast, having snacks between meals, and eating a smaller evening meal and bedtime snack. His food plan reflects these changes.

MARTY'S FOOD PLAN AND SAMPLE MENU

Calories 1750-1800

Breakfast Time: **7:00 am**

2-3	Carbohydrate Choices	1 English muffin toasted [2 choices]
		1/2 cup orange juice [1 choice]
0	Meat	
1	Fat	1 teaspoon margarine

Snack Time: **10:00 am**

1-2	Carbohydrate Choices	1 banana [2 choices]
0-1	Fat	0 added fat

Lunch Time: **12:30 pm**

2-3	Carbohydrate Choices	2 slices bread [2 choices]
		1 cup skim milk [1 choice]
1-2	Vegetable	Raw carrots
2	Meat	2 ounces lean lunch meat
1	Fat	1 teaspoon mayonnaise

Snack Time: **2:30 pm**

1-2	Carbohydrate Choices	3 squares graham crackers [1 choice]
0-1	Fat	0 added fats

Dinner Time: **6:00 pm**

3-4	Carbohydrate Choices	1 cup mashed potatoes [2 choices]
		1 cup skim milk [1 choice]
		1 small cookie [1 choice]
2-3	Vegetable	Tossed green salad
		1 cup cooked broccoli
3-4	Meat	3-4 ounces grilled chicken breast
1-2	Fat	1 teaspoon margarine
		2 tablespoons reduced-calorie dressing

Snack Time: **9:00 pm**

1-2	Carbohydrate Choices	6 cups microwave light popcorn [2]
0-1	Fat	(1 fat is hidden in the popcorn)

Chances are that you, like Marty, can identify a few behavior changes that you need to build into your food plan. The blank food plans on pages 95-96 are provided so that you can write in your planned daily servings of carbohydrate, vegetables, meat, and fat. A dietitian can help you with this, or with fine-tuning your food plan once you have the basic plan done. She or he can answer any questions you have about your plan or about specific foods. Your dietitian can also help you change your eating habits and fit your food plan into your lifestyle.

As you follow your food plan and test your blood glucose levels, you will learn more about how different foods, along with your activity level, affect your blood glucose control. You may need to adjust your number of carbohydrate choices, the spacing of food in your food plan, or your activity level to help you reach your target blood glucose goals.

Changing eating habits can be very challenging. If you want to develop a plan for improving one or more eating habits, you can use the Action Plan on page 139 (Chapter 12). Don't try to do too much all at once, though. It is better to work on just one thing at a time. Make your changes so they last a lifetime.

Key Points

- A food plan is a guide for what, when, and how much to eat to meet nutrition needs and maintain blood glucose control.
- Eating meals and snacks at regular times throughout the day helps control blood glucose levels and control appetite.
- Eating about the same amount of carbohydrate at meals and snacks each day is one of the most effective ways of controlling blood glucose levels.
- Carbohydrate counting allows flexibility in food planning.
- Serving sizes are as important as food choices for blood glucose control.
- Good nutrition is based on eating a variety of foods from all sections of the pyramid.

My Food Plan

Calories_____

Carbohydrate _____ gms (____%)   Protein _____ gms (____%)   Fat _____ gms (____%)

*Breakfast Time:*_____

_____ Carbohydrate Choices (or _____ starch _____ fruit _____ milk)

_____

_____

_____ Meat _____

_____ Fat _____

*Morning Snack Time:*_____

_____ Carbohydrate Choices (or _____ starch _____ fruit _____ milk)

_____

_____

_____   _____

*Lunch Time:*_____

_____ Carbohydrate Choices (or _____ starch _____ fruit _____ milk)

_____

_____

_____ Vegetable_____

_____ Meat _____

_____ Fat _____

*Afternoon Snack Time:*_____

_____ Carbohydrate Choices (or _____ starch _____ fruit _____ milk)

_____

_____

_____   _____

*Dinner Time:*_____

_____ Carbohydrate Choices (or _____ starch _____ fruit _____ milk)

_____

_____

_____ Vegetable_____

_____ Meat _____

_____ Fat _____

*Snack Time:*_____

_____ Carbohydrate Choices (or _____ starch _____ fruit _____ milk)

_____

_____

_____   _____

My Food Plan

Calories_____

Carbohydrate _____ gms (_____%)   Protein _____ gms (_____%)   Fat _____ gms (_____%)

*Breakfast Time:*_____

_____ Carbohydrate Choices (or _____ starch _____ fruit _____ milk)

_____

_____

_____ Meat _____

_____ Fat _____

*Morning Snack Time:*_____

_____ Carbohydrate Choices (or _____ starch _____ fruit _____ milk)

_____

_____

_____   _____

*Lunch Time:*_____

_____ Carbohydrate Choices (or _____ starch _____ fruit _____ milk)

_____

_____

_____ Vegetable_____

_____ Meat _____

_____ Fat _____

*Afternoon Snack Time:*_____

_____ Carbohydrate Choices (or _____ starch _____ fruit _____ milk)

_____

_____

_____   _____

*Dinner Time:*_____

_____ Carbohydrate Choices (or _____ starch _____ fruit _____ milk)

_____

_____

_____ Vegetable_____

_____ Meat _____

_____ Fat _____

*Snack Time:*_____

_____ Carbohydrate Choices (or _____ starch _____ fruit _____ milk)

_____

_____

_____   _____

Chapter 10

PUTTING YOUR FOOD PLAN TO WORK

In Chapter 9, you created a food plan that outlines when and how much carbohydrate, vegetables, meat, and fat to eat for meals and snacks. But there is more to food planning than that. As you put your plan into practice, you also need to know how to make food choices that will contribute to good health as well as to good blood glucose control.

Charting a Low-fat Lifestyle

Low-fat eating is not as bad as it may sound. You can still have the occasional ice-cream cone or cookie. In fact, eating low-fat foods most of the time makes it possible for you to satisfy a craving now and then without guilt. Or you may find that you even prefer to have that low-fat frozen yogurt just because it tastes good.

You can cut quite a lot of fat out of your diet without giving up favorite foods or flavor. One way is to eat smaller portions of foods you know are higher in fat. Another way is to choose low-fat foods in place of high-fat foods more often. Many low-fat food choices are available. Next time you're in the grocery store, look at the foods in your basket and check to see if there is a low-fat product that you can try as a substitute. Make the change gradually and give yourself time to adjust. Adopting this habit permanently can help you lose weight and lower your cholesterol. The shopping tips on page 98 will give you guidance for making wise choices. Copy it and take it with you to the grocery store.

ping Tips

Carbohydrate choices (Breads, Grains, Cereals, Dried Beans, Fruits, Milk)
- Choose foods that have 3 grams or less fat per serving
- Choose whole-grain breads or rolls and cereals, bagels, or English muffins
- Choose pretzels, plain popcorn, low-fat crackers, and cookies
- Compare boxed side dishes of rice, noodles, or potatoes and choose those that are lowest in fat or buy rice, noodles, or potatoes that can be prepared with less or no added fat
- Avoid doughnuts, croissants, biscuits, and most muffins
- Avoid deep-fat fried chips and snack foods
- Choose fresh, frozen, or canned fruits and vegetables without added sauces, butter, or margarine
- Choose low-fat or fat-free items like skim or 1% milk, or fat-free yogurt
- Try using evaporated skim milk as a coffee whitener

Meat and Meat Substitutes
- Choose low-fat meats such as fish, poultry, and lean beef, pork, lamb, or veal
- Choose reduced-fat or skim milk cheeses with 5 grams or less fat per ounce, such as low-fat cottage cheese, part skim mozzarella, farmer's cheese, ricotta, and monterey jack
- Choose low-fat packaged meats with 3 grams or less fat per ounce, such as packages of thinly sliced beef, chicken, turkey, and ham
- Avoid high-fat meats such as sausage, hot dogs, salamis and prime cuts of meat

Fat
- Choose a margarine that lists a liquid oil as the first ingredient
- Choose vegetable oils
- Avoid solid shortenings and butter
- Try light, low-fat, and fat-free products in place of regular products

Sweets and Desserts
- If used, substitute small amounts of sweets and desserts for carbohydrate choices
- Choose plain cookies, nonfat frozen yogurt, light ice cream, sugar-free puddings, etc.
- Limit foods high in added sweeteners and fats, such as pies, pastries, cakes, and rich desserts

Experts suggest that we eat no more than 50 to 60 grams of fat per day. It is easy to think only of added fats such as margarine, butter, oils, and salad dressings when we consider the fat we eat, but this accounts for only half the fat typically eaten in a day. The other half comes from meat and convenience or snack foods. Be sure to read the nutrition facts labels on foods to check the amount of fat.

Food preparation is another way to cut down on fat. Making small changes in the way you cook—broiling instead of frying, for instance—can make a big difference in your fat intake. You can also substitute low-fat ingredients when preparing your favorite recipes. More tips for preparing food the low-fat way are given below.

Keep in mind, too, that not all fats are created equal. Small amounts of unsaturated fats in foods are not harmful and may even offer health benefits. Saturated fat, on the other hand, con-

How to Become a Low-fat Chef

- *Bake, broil, roast, grill, microwave, steam, or poach foods rather than fry or sauté.*
- *Trim visible fat from meat before and after cooking; remove the skin from chicken before you eat it.*
- *Skim fat from broths, soups, and gravies.*
- *Use a nonstick pan or a nonstick vegetable spray instead of butter, margarine, or oil.*
- *Use herbs, non-salt seasonings, spices, and broth for flavor.*
- *Try low-cholesterol egg substitutes.*
- *Substitute two egg whites for one whole egg when baking.*
- *Use plain, low-fat yogurt, or light or fat-free sour cream or mayonnaise in place of regular sour cream or mayonnaise.*
- *Substitute liquid vegetable oil in recipes that call for solid shortening (3/4 cup oil = 1 cup shortening).*
- *Use evaporated skim milk in place of whole milk or cream when preparing cream sauces.*
- *Use evaporated skim milk as a coffee lightener in place of cream.*

tributes more to high blood cholesterol levels than unsaturated fats, and may contribute to heart disease and cancer risk.

How can you tell the difference between unsaturated and saturated fats? In general, unsaturated fats are in liquid form at room temperature, while saturated fats are solid or semi-solid at room temperature. So liquid margarine or soft margarine in a tub is a better choice than stick margarine, and liquid cooking oils (except palm and coconut oils) are a better option than solid shortening. Also, watch out for "hydrogenated oil" or "partially hydrogenated oil" when you read the Nutrition Facts labels on food packages. Hydrogen is added to some fats through a chemical process that increases the shelf life of the product. This process turns a liquid (unsaturated) fat into a more solid form (saturated). Try to limit products that list a hydrogenated oil on the label.

Eating low amounts of fat is a good idea for everyone because it helps reduce the risk of heart disease. But it's especially important for you because people with diabetes have an increased risk for developing heart disease. Remember, the changes you make for your health can be very good for others in your household, too.

Shaking the Salt Habit

All Americans are encouraged to eat less salt (sodium) because this can help prevent or control high blood pressure (hypertension). People with diabetes have even more reason to watch their table salt use and overall sodium intake because diabetes increases the likelihood that hypertension may develop. If you're overweight and have a family history of hypertension, your chances of developing high blood pressure are even greater. Although high blood pressure does not affect your blood glucose levels day to day, controlling blood pressure can lower your risk of complications from diabetes.

Sodium is a mineral that occurs naturally in foods. It is also added to many processed foods or during food preparation. Experts recommend that adults eat no more than 3000 mg of sodium per day. For people with high blood pressure, the recommended amount is 2400 mg or less sodium per day. As a reference point, there are 2300 mg of sodium in one teaspoon of table salt.

Tips for Cutting Down on Salt

- *Read food labels and choose convenience foods with 400 mg or less sodium per serving and 800 mg or less per convenience dinner or entree.*
- *Add only small amounts of salt, if any, during cooking and leave the salt shaker in the cupboard at meal times.*
- *Rinse canned foods with fresh water to reduce the sodium content.*
- *Experiment with decreasing the salt in your favorite recipes or look for low-salt recipes.*
- *Limit your use of flavorings like steak sauce, soy sauce, and Worcestershire sauce or choose low-sodium versions.*
- *Use onion powder and garlic powder in place of onion salt and garlic salt.*
- *Try fresh herbs or salt-free spice blends.*
- *Avoid high-sodium meats like bacon, ham, sausage, and lunch meats.*
- *Look for low-sodium or lower salt crackers, snacks, and soups.*

Tips for Cutting Down on Added Sugars

- *Eat fruit or low-fat or nonfat frozen yogurt for dessert.*
- *Cut back on commercial baked goods such as pastries, sweet rolls, and cookies.*
- *Reduce the amount of sugar called for in recipes. In many recipes, the sugar can be reduced by one-half to one-third without affecting the quality of the product.*
- *Add vanilla, cinnamon, or nutmeg to add flavor without adding calories.*
- *Look for sugar-free foods that have fewer than 20 calories or fewer than 5 grams carbohydrate per serving. Use these as "free" foods.*
- *Use sugar substitutes in place of sugar to sweeten beverages and foods.*

Cutting Down on Added Sugars

Although sugars have not been shown to be a risk factor for any serious health problems, it still makes good sense for everyone to use added sugars in moderation. Large amounts of added sugar provide empty calories—calories with few vitamins and minerals. Foods that contain significant amounts of added sugars are generally high in total carbohydrate and often contain large amounts of fat and calories as well. You can eat foods that contain added sugars, but be careful of the amounts and substitute them for other carbohydrate choices in your food plan.

Reading Food Labels

Food labels make it easy to determine a food's nutritional value. At a glance, you can find the serving size and the number of calories per serving. You can also learn the amounts of carbohydrate, fat, and protein provided by a serving of that food. Sodium content is also listed. The Food Label Guide on page 103 shows all the important information you can find on a food label.

Reading food labels takes the guesswork out of making healthful choices. Compare the labels on several different kinds of crackers, for instance. You will discover that the fat content of crackers can vary from zero grams to more than four grams of fat per serving. When you know this, you can then choose the crackers that have less fat in them.

Food labels are also very helpful when you are trying to cut down on sodium. Look for foods that have less than 400 mg of sodium per serving and for convenience entrees with less than 800 mg of sodium per meal.

Dining at Restaurants

It's often hard to know the fat content in foods that are prepared in a restaurant. If you're unsure, ask your server how a food is prepared before you order. You can also find clues to where the fat is when you read the menu. Table 10.1 on page 105 shows some words to watch for as you read restaurant menus.

When you eat out, order foods that are naturally lower in fat and foods that are prepared using low-fat methods. Ask for dressings, sauces, or toppings on the side so that you can decide how much of it you want to eat. Keep in mind that many restaurants are willing to prepare your food without added fat—if you ask.

Food Label Guide

Serving Size: All the information on this label is based on this portion size. If you eat double the serving size, you will consume double the calories, carbohydrate, fat, and other nutrients.

Calories: This gives the total calories per serving. Refer to the serving size to determine the calories you actually consume when you eat this food. The portion of the total calories that come from fat is also given. A good rule of thumb for convenience foods is to look for products that show one-third or fewer of the total calories coming from fat.

Total Fat: This gives the total grams of fat in a serving of that food. When buying snack foods, look for three or fewer fat grams per serving.

Saturated Fat: This shows the part of the total fat content that comes from saturated fat. Saturated fat contributes to high blood cholesterol levels. Try to use products with less than one-third of the total fat coming from saturated fat.

Sodium: This shows the amount of sodium (salt) in one serving. This is important if you are on a low-sodium diet or if you have high blood pressure. A product is considered "low-sodium" when it has less than 140 mg of sodium per serving. Avoid single serving products with more than 400 mg of sodium per serving. When buying convenience dinners, look for products with less than 800 mg of sodium in one dinner.

Total Carbohydrate: This shows the total grams of carbohydrate per serving. In your food plan, one serving of a carbohydrate food supplies 15 grams of carbohydrate (one carbohydrate choice). You must calculate the appropriate serving size for the food based on this. If a product label shows 30 grams of carbohydrate per serving, you must count it as two carbohydrate choices in your food plan.

Dietary Fiber: This shows the portion of the total carbohydrate per serving that is fiber. If you are on a high-fiber diet or want to increase your fiber intake, look for products with three or more grams of fiber per serving.

Sugar: This shows the portion of the total carbohydrate per serving that comes from sugar. This includes both natural sugar and added sugar. As a point of reference, one teaspoon of sugar has four grams of carbohydrate (15 grams equals one carbohydrate choice).

Protein: This shows the total grams of protein in one serving. Protein is an essential nutrient for growth and health.

Nutrition Facts

Serving Size 1 cup (228g)
Servings Per Container 2

Amount Per Serving

Calories 90	Calories from Fat 30

	% Daily Value*
Total Fat 3g	**5%**
Saturated Fat 0g	**0%**
Cholesterol 0mg	**0%**
Sodium 300mg	**13%**
Total Carbohydrate 13g	**4%**
Dietary Fiber 3g	**12%**
Sugars 3g	
Protein 3g	

Vitamin A 80%	•	Vitamin C 60%
Calcium 4%	•	Iron 4%

* Percent Daily Values are based on a 2,000 calorie diet. Your daily values may be higher or lower depending on your calorie needs:

	Calories:	2,000	2,500
Total Fat	Less than	65g	80g
Sat Fat	Less than	20g	25g
Cholesterol	Less than	300mg	300mg
Sodium	Less than	2,400mg	2,400mg
Total Carbohydrate		300g	375g
Dietary Fiber		25g	30g

Calories per gram:
Fat 9 • Carbohydrate 4 • Protein 4

FAST-FOOD CHOICES. There's no doubt that at times you'll find it convenient or necessary to eat fast foods. Know your food plan. Use the nutrition information the fast food chains provide to make wise choices. Chains show surprising uniformity in portion sizes and in the nutritional value of their foods. Here are a few general guidelines to help you make wise choices.

Breakfast. Start your day with plain muffins, biscuits, or toast. Request no butter and use low-sugar jam or jelly instead. Drink fruit juice and low-fat milk. Shy away from the breakfast biscuits or breakfast sandwiches, especially those on croissants. Scrambled eggs and an English muffin have less fat and sodium than many other fast-food breakfasts.

Hamburger or Fish/Chicken Sandwich. The key is to buy small. Have it plain instead of with cheese or special sauces, especially the mayonnaise-based sauces. If you've got a double-decker appetite, pile on lettuce and tomato. Choose fish and chicken sandwiches only if they're unbreaded and roasted, grilled, baked, or broiled without fat. If fried food is your only choice, choose regular coating over extra crispy varieties (which soak up more oil during cooking). Or even better, peel off the skin and lose most of the fat and excess sodium. Be sure to make full use of nonfat or low-fat extras such as salad bars to help satisfy your appetite healthfully.

French Fries. Split an order with someone else or, better yet, go with a plain baked potato or mashed potatoes. If the fries are just too tempting, limit them to a once-in-a-while treat.

Pizza. Thin-crust cheese pizza is generally the best choice when you're hungry for pizza. Choose toppings such as mushrooms, green peppers, and onions instead of pepperoni, sausage, anchovies, or extra cheese. Add a salad and the meal is even better for you!

Mexican Food. Choose tacos and tostadas, bean burritos, soft tacos, or other non-fried items. To keep the fat down, go easy on the cheese and pass on the sour cream and guacamole. Pile on extra tomatoes and salsa.

TABLE 10.1 **Fat Content Signals**

STOP!
Words that Signal High Fat Content

alfredo	fried
au gratin	in gravy, with gravy
basted	hollandaise
batter fried	marinated in oil
breaded	pan fried
buttered or buttery	pastry
cheese sauce	prime
cream sauce	rich
creamy, creamed	sauteed
deep fried	scalloped
escalloped	smothered
french fried	

GO! Words that Signal Low Fat Content

baked
broiled
char-broiled
grilled
poached
roasted
steamed
stir fried

Diabetes and Alcohol

Whether or not to drink alcoholic beverages is a personal choice. When you're deciding whether or not to have an alcoholic beverage, it helps to know how alcohol can affect you, your diabetes, and your overall health.

When a person drinks alcohol, it goes to the liver to be broken down. Alcohol is not converted to glucose, but it does provide calories that the body must use as energy or store as fat. Alcohol is a concentrated source of calories that can cause you to gain weight. And because drinking is often accompanied by eating, it may be easy to go overboard and eat too much. This can lead to high blood glucose levels.

Alcohol itself can dangerously lower blood glucose levels and can cause hypoglycemia. This is especially true if you take diabetes medications. The following guidelines are based on "occasional" use, defined as about two drinks once or twice a week:

- Never drink on an empty stomach. Always eat a reasonable amount of food to counter the blood glucose-lowering effect.
- Include both the alcohol and the food in your food plan (see Table 10.2).
- Each time, limit yourself to no more than two of the following. Each contains about the same amount of alcohol:
  - 1.5 ounces of distilled spirits (scotch, whiskey, rye, vodka, gin, cognac, rum, dry brandy)
  - 4 ounces of dry wine
  - 2 ounces of dry sherry
  - 12 ounces of beer, preferably light

Table 10.2 shows how you can include alcohol and drink mixes in your food plan. Count fruit juice drink mixes as carbohydrate choices in your food plan. However, there are a number of mixes that are calorie-free or very low in calories; they do not count as servings.

Whether it's safe for you to drink alcohol depends on your overall health, any medications you might be taking, and your diabetes control. You may want to think twice before choosing to drink alcohol in the following situations.

- If you have poor blood glucose control: Alcohol use can make it harder to get your diabetes under control.
- If you have high triglycerides: Excessive amounts of alcohol can raise your blood triglyceride level and increase your risk for heart disease.
- If you have gastritis, pancreatitis, or certain kidney and heart diseases: Alcohol can worsen these conditions. Talk with your diabetes care team about drinking alcohol if you have any of these problems.

- If you are taking prescribed or over-the-counter medications: Alcohol may interfere with your medication's effectiveness or cause a reaction. Check with your doctor or pharmacist to find out if you can safely drink alcohol while taking it.
- If you are taking glucose-lowering pills: Alcohol may react with some of the first generation glucose-lowering pills (listed on page 59) and cause unpleasant side effects. If alcohol and your glucose-lowering pills react, you will know shortly after you have the first few swallows of a drink. The reaction causes you to feel flushed or turn "beet red," have a rapid heart rate, or become dizzy or sick to your stomach. This reaction is less likely to happen with second generation glucose-lowering pills.
- If you are following a low-calorie diet: Alcohol contains a lot of empty calories. Many drinks average 100 to 300 calories each. These extra calories can make it harder to lose weight.
- If you have a history of alcohol abuse.

If you do choose to drink alcohol, do so in moderation and follow the guidelines for including it as part of your food plan.

TABLE 10.2 **Alcohol**

Alcohol and Mixes	Serving	Calories	Count as
Light beer	12 ounces	100	2 fat
Regular beer	12 ounces	150	1 carbohydrate, 2 fat
Near beer	12 ounces	60	1 carbohydrate
Liquor, any kind 86 proof	1 1/2 ounces	80 to 100	2 fat
Wine, dry	4 to 5 ounces	75 to 100	2 fat
Fruit juice	1/2 cup	60-80	1 carbohydrate
Tomato juice	1/2 cup	25	Free
Bloody Mary mix	1/2 cup	25	Free
Mineral water	any amount	0	Free
Sugar-free tonic	any amount	0	Free
Club soda	any amount	0	Free
Diet soda	any amount	0	Free

Key Points

- Choose low-fat or fat-free foods whenever possible.
- Substitute low-fat products for high-fat ingredients in recipes.
- Use low-fat cooking techniques.
- Use table salt and high-sodium foods in moderation.
- If using foods high in added sugar, substitute for carbohydrate choices.
- Read food labels and pay attention to serving sizes, fat, and calories even on low-fat and sugar-free products.
- If you drink alcohol, do so in moderation (and don't forget about the calories).

Chapter 11

DEVELOPING YOUR ACTIVITY PLAN

In Chapter 5 you learned why physical activity is so important. Now it's time to put all that knowledge to work by planning just how you are going to become and stay active.

Physical activity, as we define it, is anything that gets the large muscles in your legs and arms moving. The Activity Pyramid shows us that we have many opportunities to be active in our daily lives. You should include activities from all the sections of the pyramid for a well-rounded and active lifestyle.

You are probably already doing many things that you didn't even know could be called physical activity. Becoming more conscious of your regular activities as "physical" can help you put a little extra "oomph" into doing them. One of the greatest things about being physically active is that moving from moderate to more vigorous activity happens almost naturally. The more you do, the more you can do and the more you want to do. Walk the dog a little faster next time, feel your leg muscles working as you climb the stairs, or stay out on the dance floor for one more turn. Feel active and healthy in all that you do. And have fun!

You can probably figure out which activities from the leisure, recreational, and everyday sections of the pyramid you want to include in your plan. Use the chart on page 111 to help identify activities from these sections that you already do and those you would like to try. This information will help as you try to add more activity to your life. The rest of this chapter explains the aerobic, flexibility, and strength sections of the pyramid. These activ-

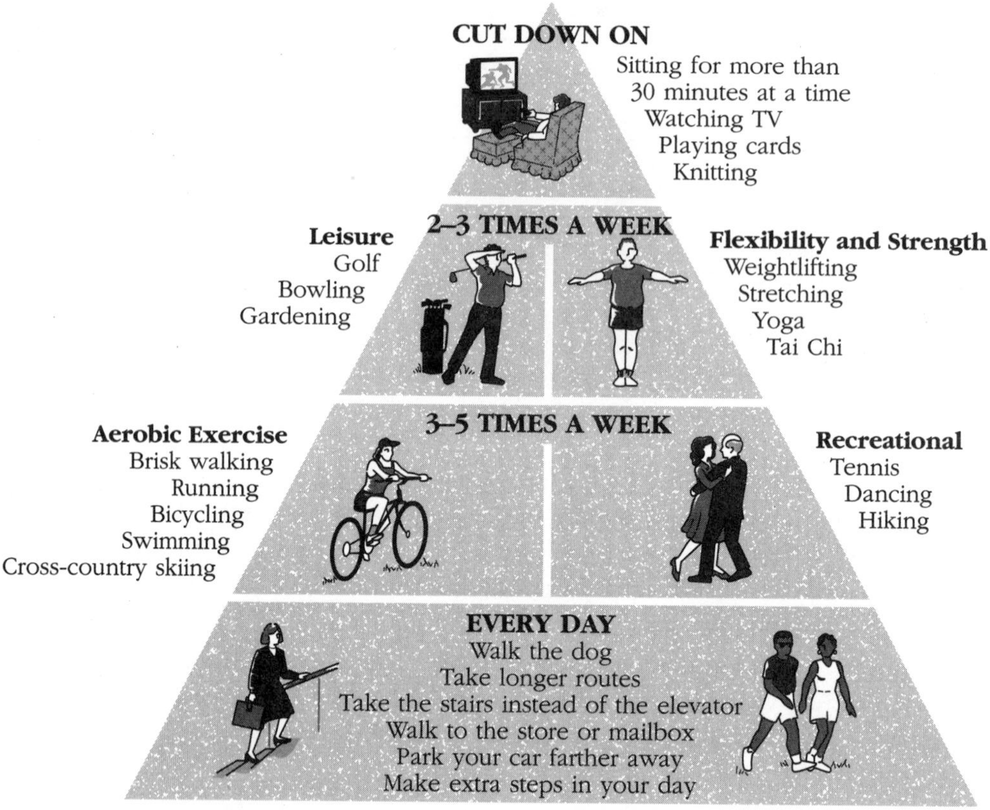

CUT DOWN ON
Sitting for more than
30 minutes at a time
Watching TV
Playing cards
Knitting

Leisure **2–3 TIMES A WEEK** **Flexibility and Strength**
Golf   Weightlifting
Bowling   Stretching
Gardening   Yoga
Tai Chi

Aerobic Exercise **3–5 TIMES A WEEK** **Recreational**
Brisk walking   Tennis
Running   Dancing
Bicycling   Hiking
Swimming
Cross-country skiing

EVERY DAY
Walk the dog
Take longer routes
Take the stairs instead of the elevator
Walk to the store or mailbox
Park your car farther away
Make extra steps in your day

FIGURE 11.1 **Activity Pyramid**
Adapted from *The Activity Pyramid,* © 1995 Institute for Research and Education
HealthSystem Minnesota

ities are the backbone of your active lifestyle and will do the most
to improve your heart health, level of fitness, and diabetes control.

Aerobic vs. Anaerobic Activity

Aerobic activity is at the center of any program aimed at improving health and physical fitness. "Aerobic" refers to "air." The muscles, including the heart, require a steady supply of oxygen to continue working at an increased level for any length of time. Aerobic activities are those that get your heart rate up to a comfortable working level and keep it there. This kind of activity is

Put a check by the activities you already do or would like to try. You may write in any that are not listed here. Circle those that you participate in regularly (at least once a week, or as a regularly scheduled activity).

Leisure
- ❑ Golf
- ❑ Bowling
- ❑ Softball
- ❑ Yard work
- ❑ Gardening
- ❑ Shopping
- ❑ Others:

_____

_____

_____

_____

Recreational
- ❑ Hiking
- ❑ Dancing
- ❑ Canoeing
- ❑ Tai Chi
- ❑ Walking
- ❑ Swimming
- ❑ Tennis
- ❑ Bicycling
- ❑ In-line skating
- ❑ Jogging
- ❑ Others:

_____

_____

_____

Every day
- ❑ Walking the dog
- ❑ Using the stairs
- ❑ Walking to errands
- ❑ Parking further away
- ❑ Housework
- ❑ Morning stretches
- ❑ Daily stretch breaks
- ❑ Walking around workplace during breaks
- ❑ Others:

_____

_____

_____

excellent for weight control because it burns fat. Few daily activities are truly aerobic. It is usually necessary to plan for and make an effort to include aerobic activity in our lives.

"Anaerobic" means "without air." Anaerobic activities are generally shorter in duration and more intense than aerobic activities, or they may require you to be active in short bursts followed by periods of rest. The muscles cannot get enough oxygen to do anaerobic activities for sustained periods of time. Anaerobic activities, especially flexibility and strength exercises, are a very important part of your activity plan.

Table 11.1 shows the differences between aerobic and anaerobic activities and some examples of each. Include both types of activity in your activity plan. Both will lower your blood glucose, but you will receive the greatest overall health benefit from aerobic activity. We will discuss aerobic activity first. Flexibility and strength activities (anaerobic) are discussed later in this chapter.

TABLE 11.1 **Aerobic and Anaerobic Activity**

	Aerobic	**Anaerobic**
Characteristics	With oxygen 20 minutes or more in duration Burns fat more than carbohydrate Uses large muscles (arms and legs) Continuous movement Gives greatest health benefits Lowers LDL and total cholesterol Raises HDL cholesterol Helps control weight	Without oxygen Less than 20 minutes in duration Burns carbohydrate more than fat Start and stop movements Includes flexibility and strength exercises
Examples	Walking Bicycling, regular or stationary Swimming laps Aerobic dance class Marching in place Armchair aerobics Water aerobics Cross-country skiing Ski machine Stair-climbing machine	Lifting weights Sit-ups Push-ups Stretching Walking up stairs Most team sports Gardening or yard work Housework

Aerobic Activity

To be sure you get the most from aerobic activity, you must pay attention to three things: frequency, duration, and intensity. Frequency means how many times each week you do an activity or exercise session. Duration means how long each activity session lasts. Intensity refers to how hard you are actually working during the activity.

This may sound like a lot of work already—and you haven't even started exercising yet! It's really not that hard or complicated. Table 11.2 outlines the goals and recommendations for the frequency, duration, and intensity of aerobic activity. Set your goals based on your current level of activity and fitness. If you are inactive, start with the recommendations given in the table and gradually increase your activity level as you feel comfortable.

TABLE 11.2 **Goals and Recommendations for Aerobic Activity**

	Recommendations	Goal
Frequency	Start with 1 to 2 sessions more per week than you currently do.	3 to 7 times a week
Duration	Start with 10 minutes per session for one week. Increase by 5 to 10 minutes per session each week until you reach your goal.	20 to 45 minutes per session
Intensity	Start at an easy or moderate perceived exertion level and increase intensity over time.	Moderate to somewhat hard perceived exertion. (see Table 11.3)

It is common for people to try to do too much too fast. Somehow we feel that we'll get in shape faster if we just work harder. Nothing could be further from the truth. Working too hard (intensity) or too much (frequency) or for too long (duration) causes most people to "burn out" on their activity. It just isn't fun so they stop doing it. Remember, too, that it can be dangerous to exercise beyond your fitness level. Don't make this mistake. It is best and easiest to increase frequency or duration first and then work on intensity goals.

See your physician before starting an activity program if you are over age 40 and inactive, or if you have uncontrolled high blood pressure or heart trouble.

Checking Your Intensity

You can keep the intensity of your activity within a safe and comfortable range by doing two things: listening to your body (perceived exertion) and checking your heart rate. Always take time to check your intensity as you do your activity. You want to be sure you are working hard enough to get the benefits of the activity, but not so hard that you cause more harm than good.

PERCEIVED EXERTION. Checking your heart rate (checking your pulse) is commonly used to measure intensity, but it may not always be the best way to tell how hard you are exercising. Instead, you can determine how hard your heart is working by "listening" to your body during your activity. This is an especially effective method for many people with diabetes because nerve problems (neuropathy) can cause your pulse to be an unreliable indicator of how hard your heart is working. This is also true for people who take medications called beta blockers for blood pressure or heart disease, since the medications are used to keep the heart rate lowered.

Listening to your body means noticing how your body feels during an activity. Moderate aerobic activity will cause you to breathe deeper and faster than usual. However, it should not cause you to huff and puff. If it's a struggle to talk during your activity, slow down. You are working too hard. Notice how you feel as you exercise and compare it to the descriptions in the perceived exertion scale (Table 11.3). For a safe yet vigorous workout, stay in the moderate to somewhat hard range.

In short, push yourself, but stay within your comfort range. If something hurts, don't do it.

HEART RATE. Even when you are using perceived exertion to measure your intensity, it's still a good idea to check your pulse in the middle of each activity session so you can be sure you are in your recommended range. Table 11.4 lists general target ranges for

TABLE 11.3 **Perceived Exertion Scale**

Nothing	Easy	Moderate	Somewhat Hard	Hard	Very Hard
Normal breathing	Breathing a little faster	Breathing faster and deeper	Breathing heavier but able to talk	Breathing heavy, barely able to talk	Panting and unable to talk
No unusual muscle activity	Muscles warming up	Muscles feel like they are working	Muscles feel strong and able to go on	Muscles feel tired, barely able to go on	Muscles feel weak

How to Take Your Pulse

You can feel your pulse by placing your index and middle fingers on one of two locations. The first spot is at the base of your wrist, about an inch below the bone on the thumb side of your hand. You can also find your pulse at the side of your neck about halfway between the point of your chin and your ear.

After you find your pulse, look at the second hand of a watch or a stopwatch so you can measure exactly ten seconds. Beginning with zero, count the number of beats you feel in ten seconds. Compare the number of beats to the target heart rate shown for your age in Table 11.4.

people of different ages. Your target heart rate may be different from these ranges, especially if you have heart disease or if you are just starting an exercise plan. Ask your doctor or diabetes care team what an appropriate range is for you.

Your pulse will tell you how fast your heart is beating. Take your pulse after ten to fifteen minutes of doing your activity. This gives your body enough time to get "up to speed." If you intend to continue your activity after taking your pulse, try not to stop entirely as you do it. Your heart rate may fall and you'll have to build up to your working level again.

If your heart rate is below the range for your age, you'll need to speed up a little. Sometimes using your arms a little more vigorously, such as pumping them when you walk, will be enough to push your heart rate up into your range. If your heart rate is too high, slow down. You might let your arms hang still for a few moments, then slowly begin using them again.

TABLE 11.4 **Target Heart Rates for Aerobic Activity**

Age	Beats per 10 seconds
30	19-24
35	19-23
40	18-23
45	18-22
50	17-21
55	17-21
60	16-20
65	16-19
70	15-19
75	15-18
80	14-18
85	14-17

Warm-up and Cool-down Activities

Your heart and the other muscles in your body do not like to be jolted from inactivity into vigorous action. Starting your activity without a proper warm-up can cause muscles to be sore afterward or, worse, can cause injury. Warm-up activities help your body move gradually from resting to working. Similarly, cool-down activities help move your body back to its resting state.

Ready your body for aerobic activity by doing a slow version of the activity for five to fifteen minutes. For instance, if you walk, warm up with a slow walk using your arms; if you bike, warm up by pedaling slowly. These warm-up activities raise your heart rate gradually.

You may want to follow this short warm-up with a few gentle stretches to loosen your muscles and prepare them for more movement. Look at the next section in this chapter for examples of stretches you might do. Hold each stretch for 20 to 30 seconds and don't bounce. Just go as far as you comfortably can while getting a good stretching feeling in the muscle you are working. The warm-up is a time for easy stretches.

After you finish your activity, allow your heart rate to return to its pre-activity rate by cooling down. Like the warm-up, cool-down movements can be as simple as a slower version of your aerobic activity. Take your pulse after five to fifteen minutes to check that your heart rate has returned to its resting rate. A resting heart rate is usually under 95 beats per minute. Check yours anytime during the normal activity of your day and note it so you have a reference point.

Follow your cool-down period with a few stretches. You will be able to stretch more fully after your aerobic activity, when your muscles are warm and loosened.

Flexibility and Strength Activities

Aerobic activity is very important, but staying fit and healthy requires more. We also need to keep our bodies flexible and our

To Help You Lose Weight

Aerobic activity is one of the best ways to lose weight because the body burns stored fat as fuel. Aerobic activities are even more effective for weight loss when combined with better food habits, such as eating smaller portions and eating less fat. You will get the best results if you are continuously active for at least 20 to 30 minutes at a "somewhat hard" perceived exertion (see Table 11.3 on page 114). Try to do an aerobic activity four to six times a week if you want to lose weight.

muscles toned. Strong and flexible muscles give our bodies freedom of movement and the ability to protect itself from injury. You can do a number of activities to improve your flexibility and strength.

FLEXIBILITY ACTIVITIES. Muscles and connective tissue tend to tighten up as we get older. This tightness can cause discomfort and can limit movement. The best way to stay flexible or to increase flexibility is through slow stretching. As you try some of the stretches presented here, be sure to stretch as far as you can, but not to the point of pain. Gradually these stretches will increase your flexibility. They will also help to protect your body from low back pain and injuries.

Overhead Stretch
- Stand comfortably.
- Reach up with both arms as high as you can.
- Hold your stomach in, push your chest out, and bring your shoulders back.
- Lift your heels up and stand on your toes.
- Hold stretch for 10 to 20 counts.
- Repeat two to three times.

Calf Stretch
- Facing the wall, place both hands on the wall at shoulder height.
- Bring one foot forward, bending the knee.
- Place your other foot behind you, toes facing forward, straightening the leg and pushing the heel to the floor.
- Hold stretch for 10 to 20 counts.
- Repeat with your other leg.

Thigh Stretch
- Face the wall with your feet shoulder width apart.
- Place left hand on the wall for support.
- With your right hand, grasp your right ankle and pull it toward your buttocks.

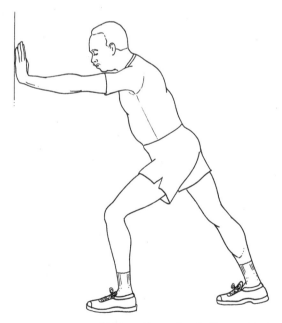

FIGURE 11.1 **Calf Stretch—Flexibility Activity**

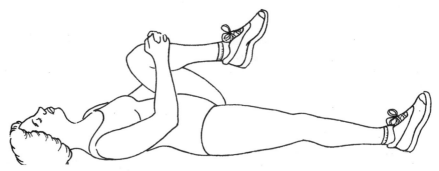

FIGURE 11.2 **Lower Back Stretch—Flexibility Activity**

- Keep bent knee facing toward the floor and close to the knee of your straight leg.
- Hold stretch for 10 to 20 counts.
- Repeat with your other leg.

Lower Back Stretch
- Lie on your back with legs extended.
- Bend one knee and bring it as close to your chest as possible.
- Hold the stretch for 10 to 20 counts.
- Repeat with your other leg.

Hamstring Stretch
- Lie on your back with legs extended.
- Bend one knee and bring it toward your chest.
- Supporting your thigh with your hands, straighten your leg toward the ceiling.
- Stretch only as far as you comfortably can.
- Hold the stretch for 10 to 20 counts.
- Repeat with your other leg.

STRENGTH ACTIVITIES. Activities that build and maintain strength improve the condition of muscles and keep them toned. Strength activities are essential for maintaining range of motion in limbs and joints and for improving balance and coordination. The following exercises are examples of strength activities.

Arm Extensions
- Stand with your legs shoulder width apart and arms extended to the sides at chest level. This is your starting position.

- Slowly bring arms up over your head and then lower them to starting position.
- Slowly lower arms straight down to your sides, feeling the tension as you pull down. Return to starting position.
- Slowly lift your arms forward in front of your body to shoulder height.
- Slowly reach your arms around to extend behind your back. Return to starting position.
- Repeat entire cycle three times.

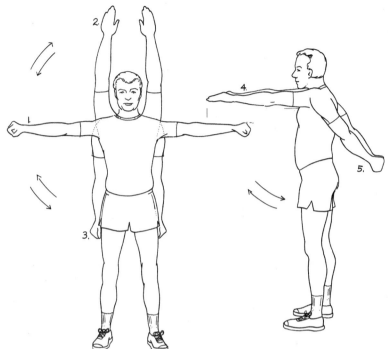

FIGURE 11.3 **Arm Extensions—Strength Activity**

Pelvic Tilt

- Lie on your back with your knees bent, feet flat on the floor.
- Concentrate on the lower part of your back; push it down into the floor.
- Hold for 10 to 20 counts.
- Release and allow your back to come up off the floor.
- Repeat five times.

Curl-Ups

- Lie on your back with your knees bent, feet flat on the floor. Rest your hands by your sides.
- Lift your head up by tightening your stomach muscles and bring your chin toward your chest.
- Hold for five seconds.
- Repeat as many times as you comfortably can. (After you gain strength, try lifting your upper back and shoulders as well as your head.)

Side Leg Lifts

- Lie on your right side with your right knee slightly bent for support. Keep your knees and hips facing forward.

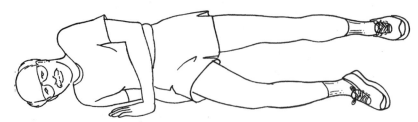

FIGURE 11.4 **Side Leg Lifts—Strength Activity**

• Place your left hand out in front of your body.
• Slowly lift your extended left leg upward four to six inches. Do not try to lift your leg higher.
• Hold for three to five seconds, then slowly lower your leg.
• Lift two to five times. Repeat with your right leg.

Back Leg Swings

• Stand with your hands against a wall for support. Your hands should be at eye level.
• Slowly lift your right leg back, keeping your knee straight. Feel your hamstring and buttock tighten.
• Hold for three to five seconds, and return your leg to a standing position.
• Lift two to five times. Repeat with your left leg.

Get Fit While You Sit

Seated activities are a good choice if you have a hard time standing or walking, if you've just started exercising, or if you don't want to jar your joints or bones. We call these activities "armchair activities." Armchair activities can be aerobic (marching in place) or anaerobic (stretching).

Several armchair aerobic and stretching activities are presented here. While you do armchair activities, keep your back straight and continue to breathe deeply. Stop if you feel any pain, if you have shortness of breath, or if you feel faint. Tell your physician if you have any of these signs while doing your activity.

Mix and match armchair leg and arm movements to create your own aerobic activity. An example of this would be to sit and move your legs in a marching motion as you circle your arms forward

and backward (see Figure 11.5). Armchair aerobics can be followed by armchair stretches to help you cool down and improve
muscle flexibility. Choose two or three armchair stretching exercises to complete your activity.

Armchair Aerobics

Try to keep up your aerobic activity for at least ten minutes. You
can increase the duration as your fitness level improves.

LEG MOVEMENTS

Marching
- Sit with both feet flat on the floor, about eight to ten inches
  apart.
- Keeping knees bent, lift your right foot three to six inches off
  the floor, then set it down.
- Repeat with your left foot. Alternate legs in a rhythmic, marching motion.

Flutter Kicks
- Sit and extend your legs by straightening them slightly.
- Lift your feet three to six inches from the floor.
- Kick your right leg slightly upward, then downward from the
  knee. Lightly tap the floor with
  your toe on the downswing.
  Repeat with the left leg.
- Kick alternate legs quickly, as if
  swimming.

Side Step
- Sit with both feet flat on the
  floor, about eight to ten inches
  apart.
- Lift your right leg and move it
  over to touch your right toe to
  your left heel. Avoid twisting
  your ankle when you do this.
- Lift and move your right foot
  back to its starting position.

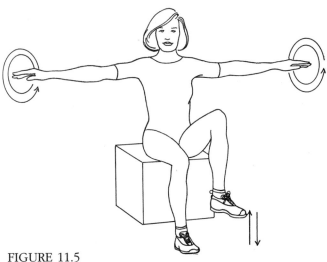

FIGURE 11.5
Marching Legs and Arm Circles—Armchair Aerobics

- Repeat the movement with your left leg, touching your left toe to your right heel.
- Continue the movement, alternating legs quickly and rhythmically.

Alternate Toe Taps
- Sit with both feet flat on the floor, about eight to ten inches apart.
- Lift and reach your right foot forward about six inches and tap the floor with your toe, then bring your foot back to the original position.
- Repeat with left foot. Alternate legs quickly and rhythmically.

Side-to-Side Leg Sways
- Sit with feet flat on the floor and close together.
- Lift both feet and move them about six inches to the left. Tap the floor lightly with your toes.
- In a continuous motion, swing your feet back to the right, about six inches past the starting point, and tap the floor again with your toes.
- Continue swaying feet from side to side, touching toes to the floor with each swing.

ARM MOVEMENTS

Arm Circles
- Hold arms out to sides at shoulder level, palms facing downward. Keep arms straight, but avoid "locking" your elbows.
- Circle arms forward or backward, making circles as small or as large as is comfortable.

Arm Pushes
- Hold your arms out to the sides at shoulder level, palms facing forward. Keep your arms straight, but avoid locking elbows.
- Move arms forward with short, swift pushing motions.
- You can also do this exercise with an upward, downward, or backward pushing motion. Your palms should face the direction you push in.

Crawl or Breaststroke
- *The Crawl:* Move arms over your head and forward in the conventional swimming motion.

- *The Breaststroke:* Begin with arms close to your body, elbows bent and hands close together at your chest. Push arms forward, then out to the sides with a smooth, circular motion. Bring hands together again and repeat.

Bicep curls
- Hold your arms out straight to the sides at shoulder level, palms facing upward.
- Bend your elbows so that arms form 90-degree angles, your upper arms parallel to the floor.
- Lower arms back to straight position and repeat.

Armchair Stretching Exercises

When stretching, never hold your breath; breathe deeply and evenly. Stretch as far as you comfortably can, and try to hold the stretches for at least 10 to 20 counts.

Neck Stretches
- Sit with your hands in your lap.
- Slowly drop your head to one side and hold for ten counts.
- Repeat on the other side.
- Repeat three times for each side.

Shoulder Rolls
- Slowly roll your shoulders backward in a circle ten times.
- Reverse direction, slowly rolling shoulders forward ten times.

Overhead Stretches
- Place your hands on your shoulders.
- Slowly reach one hand toward the ceiling, fully extending your arm.
- Slowly return the hand to the shoulder.
- Alternate arms, repeating ten times with each arm.

Lateral Stretches
- Sit with your left hand in your lap.
- Reach with right hand over your head and toward the ceiling over your left shoulder.
- Repeat with left arm over your right shoulder, resting the right hand in your lap.
- Repeat ten times with each arm, alternating arms.

Leg Stretches
- Slowly lift one leg until it is parallel to floor and point the toes.
- Hold for five counts.
- Flex the foot and hold for five more counts.
- Repeat ten times with each leg, alternating legs.

Knee Pulls
- Clasp your hands around the front of one knee.
- Slowly pull the knee toward your chest.
- Hold for five counts.
- Repeat ten times with each knee, alternating knees.

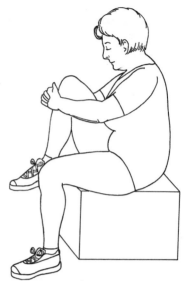

FIGURE 11.6 **Knee Pulls—Armchair Stretch Activity**

Ankle Circles
- Lift one foot slightly off the floor.
- Rotate the foot and draw a circle in the air with the toes.
- Complete the circle ten times.
- Repeat with the other foot.

Ankle Point and Flex
- Lift one leg slightly off the floor.
- Slowly point your toe, then slowly bring the toes back until the foot is flexed.
- Complete ten point and flex movements.
- Repeat with the other leg.

Your Activity Plan

Now that you know the things you need to include in an activity session, you can start putting your plan together. For each aerobic activity session, include a warm-up time (5 to 15 minutes); an aerobic activity (20 to 45 minutes); and a cool-down time (5 to 10 minutes). Strive to do an aerobic activity at least three times a week.

Try to do stretching (5 to 10 minutes) and strengthening activities (10 to 30 minutes) at least twice a week. These activities can be done in conjunction with your aerobic activity as described in this chapter or at other times. Just be sure to warm up before any type of physical activity.

STEP 1 The first thing you need to do is identify the activities that you may want to do. List the aerobic, stretching, and strengthening activities you do or would like to do in the space provided. Choose from those discussed in this chapter (Table 11.1 on page 112 shows aerobic activities) or include others of your own. You can then use these choices to develop your own personal activity sessions.

Parts of an Activity Session

Warm-up	5 to 15 min.	before any type of activity
Aerobic	20 to 45 min.	at least three times a week
Cool-down	5 to 10 min.	after any type of activity
Stretching	5 to 10 min.	at least twice a week
Strength	10 to 30 min.	at least twice a week

Aerobic Activities I Like/Want to Do:

_____

_____

_____

Stretching Activities I Like/Want to Do:

_____

_____

_____

Strengthening Activities I Like/Want to Do:

_____

_____

_____

STEP 2 Now it's time for you to plan an activity session. Choose one aerobic activity, two or three stretching activities, and one or two strengthening activities from your lists. Write them in the chart below. A few sample sessions are shown on the next page.

Remember to start with what is comfortable for you, and don't try to do too much too fast. You may wish to develop a few different activity sessions to try. The important thing is to do something—and to keep doing it! Research shows that the benefits of activity start to diminish after only three days of inactivity. Consistency is more important than intensity.

Personal Activity Session One

Program Part	Duration	Activity
Warm-up	5 minutes	
Aerobic	15 to 20 minutes	
Cool-down	5 minutes	
Stretching	Until done	
Strength	Until done	

Personal Activity Session Two

Program Part	Duration	Activity
Warm-up	5 minutes	
Aerobic	15 to 20 minutes	
Cool-down	5 minutes	
Stretching	Until done	
Strength	Until done	

Sample Session: Walking or Marching

Program Part	Duration	Activity
Warm-up	5 minutes	March in place and move arms up and down
Aerobic	15 to 20 minutes	Walk or march at moderate pace and move arms
Cool-down	5 minutes	Side step right and left; back and forth
Stretching	5 minutes	Choose and do 2 leg stretches and 2 arm stretches
Strength	Until done	10 curl ups

Sample Session: Bicycling

Program Part	Duration	Activity
Warm-up	5 minutes	Pedal slowly
Aerobic	15 to 20 minutes	Pedal at a moderate pace
Cool-down	5 minutes	Pedal slowly
Stretching	Until done	Choose and do 3 leg stretches
Strength	Until done	25 arm circles forward, 25 arm circles backward

Sample Session: Seated

Program Part	Duration	Activity
Warm-up	5 minutes	March legs up and down while doing bicep curls
Aerobic	15 to 20 minutes	Continue leg movements; do arm circles
Cool-down	5 minutes	Slow down arm and leg movements
Stretching	Until done	Choose and do 3 seated stretches
Strength	Until done	Lift and lower each leg 20 times

STEP 3 It's easy to allow busy schedules and distractions to inter-fere with an activity plan, so you need to think about when you can do your activity and schedule it. You can use the Activity Plan calendar on page 128 to do this (you may want to photocopy it for use in future months). If you already use a personal calendar or day planner, you may also want to write your planned activi-ties in that calendar to avoid conflicts.

Consider carefully what times of the day and which days of the week are best for your activity. At the beginning of each week,

Activity Plan

	SUN	MON	TUES	WED	THUR	FRI	SAT
Sample	*Brisk walk with dog 8-8:30 am*		*Aerobics class 6-7 pm*		*Bowling 7-8 pm*	*Lunchtime walk 12-12:30 pm*	
Week 1							
Week 2							
Week 3							
Week 4							
Week 5							
Week 6							

look at your other plans and commitments for that week and decide when you could fit activity sessions into your schedule. Then write the activity you plan to do and when you plan to do it on the calendar. A sample week is shown on the calendar.

After you complete each scheduled activity session, draw an X through it—and feel good about yourself. If you don't complete a session, circle it. At the end of the month, look over your calendar and try to spot patterns that can help you plan future activities. For example, if you schedule several after-dinner walking sessions throughout the month and keep nearly all of them, that time slot will probably work on an ongoing basis. If, however, you find that you are missing many of your scheduled activity times, you will have to make some adjustments. Remember to check with your physician or diabetes care team before starting your activity program if you are over age 40 and inactive, if you have uncontrolled high blood pressure, or if you have heart trouble.

Hypoglycemia

If you take glucose-lowering pills or insulin to treat your diabetes, physical activity can sometimes make your blood glucose level drop too low. If your blood glucose falls below 80 mg/dl (4.4 mM/L) while you are active, you may begin to feel shaky, dizzy, and sweaty. These are symptoms of *hypoglycemia*. (You can read more about hypoglycemia on page 78.) You can help prevent hypoglycemia by testing your blood glucose level before beginning any physical activity. If your blood glucose level is below 100 mg/dl (5.5 mM/L) just before an activity that will last more than 30 minutes, eat a snack (15 grams of carbohydrate).

Always carry a carbohydrate food with you when you exercise; the Hypoglycemia Safety Kit offers some suggestions. If you begin to feel early symptoms of hypoglycemia, stop your activity and eat your carbohydrate food. It's also wise to wear a medical ID bracelet when you exercise. Keep track of any times you become hypoglycemic during or after exercise. If this happens more than two or three times a week, talk to your diabetes care team. They may advise you to space your food differently throughout the day or to adjust your diabetes medication.

Hypoglycemia Safety Kit

Keep one or two of the following foods with you when you exercise:

- *3–4 glucose tablets (each tablet contains 4–5 grams of carbohydrate)*
- *1 small box or 2 tablespoons raisins*
- *2 large sugar cubes or 5 small sugar cubes*
- *6 or 7 hard candies*

Key Points

- Any physical activity can help control your diabetes and improve your health.
- Aerobic activity is the cornerstone of physical fitness.
- Include flexibility and strength activities in your program.
- Start slowly and gradually increase how long and how often you are active.
- Check the intensity of your activity by listening to your body or taking your pulse. Don't overdo it.
- If you take glucose-lowering pills or inject insulin, carry some carbohydrate food with you when you exercise.
- See your physician before starting an activity program if you are over age 40 and inactive, or if you have uncontrolled high blood pressure or heart trouble.

Chapter 12

LEARNING HOW TO CHANGE

We live in a health-conscious society that reminds us to watch our blood pressure, lose some weight, quit smoking, stay out of the sun, and so on. All of this is good advice. Ironically, the same society that promotes healthful choices also promotes instant gratification—from fast food meals to rapid weight loss. These are difficult messages to balance when you're trying to make healthful changes that will help you manage your diabetes. Most of us realize that making lifestyle changes is neither quick nor easy. We may make some progress, but then we lapse back into the old behavior. Then we try again. Learning how to change is a *process*, and it takes time to succeed.

If you look closely at people who are successfully managing their diabetes, there are many things at work. They're usually both motivated and hopeful that they can reach their goals. They also often have a network of supportive friends and health care professionals, or they seek out a support system. Most importantly, they set realistic goals and develop a plan to reach those goals.

This chapter gives you an opportunity to examine the different phases of behavior change, especially as it relates to diabetes management. Change need not—and probably should not—be dramatic. Instead, change is gradual and is accomplished through making many small decisions that lead to overall success.

Acknowledging the Need to Change

When you don't recognize a problem, you can't solve it. For example, if you don't believe diabetes is serious, you may not do much to take care of it. People around you—your spouse, friends, or diabetes care team—may express concern, and you may tell yourself, "Other people think I need to make changes, but I think they're overreacting." Even as you think this, something inside may be telling you that they are right.

Desired change cannot take place until you honestly and consciously believe that it is needed. Only then will you have the motivation to take steps toward actually making a change. This is true in all areas of life, not just in managing your diabetes.

This stage is often marked by ambivalent feelings. You know it would probably be better if you made a change—if you ate fewer fatty foods, for instance—but you just don't feel like it or it seems too hard, maybe even impossible. These are natural reactions that are part of the change process. After all, making lifestyle changes is challenging and we often find ways to talk ourselves out of doing things that are hard. This is a problem because it can stop you from doing what you know is best for your health.

To move through this stage of change, you need to identify the feelings and internal messages that are getting in your way. This can be difficult because your surface resistance may not be the real issue. Behind thoughts such as, "It just isn't worth it to exercise—I tried it before and nothing happened," may be deeper messages like, "I can't do it. I'm weak willed. I will fail." It is only when you know and understand the true source of your resistance that you can begin to work through it. In time, you can change your internal messages to be positive and supportive of your desire to change.

If you find yourself in this stage, try to identify what is hindering you. Reflect on how you feel and why you might be reluctant to make changes. To begin, ask yourself:

- How do I feel about having diabetes?
- Am I afraid of change? Why?
- Do I believe it simply doesn't matter?
- Do I lack self confidence?

Your answers to these questions will help you begin to move through this stage of change. You may also gather more information about diabetes and making changes through books, videos, and lectures. Your diabetes care team is also a good source of information and support.

Getting Ready to Change

The next stage in the change process is a period of preparation because, even though you may believe that you need to change, you may not be ready to do it. You may not know quite what to do to make the needed change, or you may lack motivation. This stage is marked by thoughts such as, "I know I need to make a change, but how do I know it's worth the effort?" or "I want to make this behavior change, but I'm not sure how to start."

Proper preparation is essential for successful change. You need to be ready, both psychologically and physically, to start out on the right track and to stay your course. Even when you are well-prepared to make a change, you can expect challenges and lapses along the way. When you are not prepared, you may put a lot of effort into an ill-fated plan that will only cause you to become discouraged when it doesn't work.

Psychological preparation includes having a strong belief that the change can be made and being committed to making it happen. Belief and commitment will help you deal with feelings of ambivalence and resistance, and will help you continue on your course. These feelings tend to creep back again and again throughout the change process, challenging your resolve. One strategy for preparing yourself psychologically for change is to make a contract with yourself such as the Action Plan on page 139. When you think through your plan clearly, write it out, and sign your name to it, you make it "real." It is no longer something you *might* do; it is something you promised yourself you *will* do.

Physical preparation may include gathering information, resources, and support to help you get started on the right track. You need to be reasonably sure that what you do—the change you make—is going to produce the desired results, and you need to "stack the deck" in your favor by creating a personal plan for success. For instance, if you want to begin an activity program that will help you lose weight, you need to know what kind of activity to do, how often you should do it, and how "hard" you should do it. You also need to know things about yourself: Would you rather do a solo activity or do something with a group? Do you need a set schedule or something more flexible? And so on.

The preparation stage is a good time to talk to other people about the changes you want to make. You can talk to people who have diabetes to learn about their trials and successes. You can talk to your diabetes care team to ask questions and get information or ideas. And you can talk to your family and friends to ask for their support. All of these people can be a great source of encouragement to you and can help hold you accountable for the changes you plan to make.

This is also a good time to do some self-evaluation. Some questions you could ask yourself are:

- What can I do to make a difference in how I feel both physically and emotionally?
- Who is available to help me?
- Can I make a modest change in my eating or exercise habits?
- How will making changes affect my life?
- What is really important to me?

All of your preparations for change work together to increase your motivation to take action. Take the time you need to get ready. The changes you make to help manage your diabetes are life-long changes. And change takes time.

Taking Action

This stage is very obvious. You have a plan to accomplish your needed change and are consciously following it. You are making different choices. This stage is marked by making changes in your environment or in your reactions to your environment that support your needed change. This includes removing temptations to return to your old behavior. The following strategies can help you succeed in this stage.

- *Self-monitor by keeping food, exercise, and blood glucose records.* People with diabetes who participate in behavior change programs report that this is very helpful. Monitoring acts as a sort of conscience to keep you on track with your new behavior. It also shows you immediate results for your effort.

- *Change your environment.* This sometimes requires the cooperation of family and friends, but they will often benefit by going along with you. For example, don't allow high-fat snacks in the house, set a specific time to eat meals and snacks, and set aside a time and place for exercise.

- *Substitute a healthy behavior for your old habit.* Do you often meet a friend for coffee and dessert? Decide to go walking, golfing, or shopping instead. Do you find yourself eating snacks when you watch a favorite television show? Plan to have a low-fat snack that is part of your food plan, such as unbuttered popcorn, a sugar-free popsicle, or two small cookies.

- *Outsmart the problem.* Before the "testing" time comes, think about situations that always have been a challenge to you and anticipate how you might react the next time. For example, if you know that past social situations have led to overeating and you have a party to attend soon, anticipate the problem and plan ways to handle it differently. Plan one: Eat a snack to curb your appetite before you go. Plan two: Fill your plate with free foods or foods from your food plan when you attend the party. Plan three: Stay on the other side of the room from the food table.

- *Reward yourself.* Good health may be the natural reward for changing your habits, but sometimes it helps to do something more. Did you work in your garden instead of watching television? Great! Buy yourself a new garden tool! Think about ways to reward yourself when you reach your short-term goals. Have a grand celebration when you reach your long-term goals!

Reaching and Maintaining Personal Goals

Think about when you first began to read, play a musical instrument, or play a sport. Unless you were a natural genius, you had to practice. You started with small steps and you kept getting better and better, though sometimes you had to go back a few steps and do them again.

Making lifestyle changes is much the same. Everyone who attempts to change a behavior finds maintaining the behavior a challenge. But every time you take a new step or stumble, you learn from that experience. Each step in this process helps you gain more skill and confidence in your ability to do something new.

As you continue down this path of change, be aware that the pitfalls that were part of your life before can still be a problem. You may still catch yourself falling back into old patterns of behavior. In order to maintain your lifestyle changes, try to follow these helpful strategies:

- *Learn stress management strategies.* Stressful situations are the number-one reason people go back to old behaviors. If you're feeling very upset about something or have just had a bad day, don't reach for high-fat food! Now is the time to exercise, eat a piece of fruit, write in a journal, or talk to a friend. Train yourself to handle daily stresses in ways that will not defeat your health goals.
- *Visit regularly with your diabetes care team.* They will help you assess how you're doing and give you encouragement. They can also offer you tips for how to solve frustrating problems.
- *Learn to cope with relapse.* For example if you *do* eat too much at a party, don't tell yourself that you've "blown it" and that you cannot change. No one is perfect, and an occasional lapse is inevitable. Forgive yourself and get right back on your food plan the next day. If you need to make up for the extra eating, add extra time to your exercise session. You're still much further along than you were when you started. If despite your best efforts you find yourself relapsing often, you may need to redesign your goal to be more realistic. You may also need to do more research about the problem before you take action again.

Developing an Action Plan

To develop an action plan, start with one area of change and set short- and long-term goals. For example, your long-term goal may be to follow your food plan every day, or to do an aerobic activity for thirty minutes three days a week, or to test your blood glucose regularly. In the short term, you might plan to follow your food plan two days out of the week (including a weekend day), or to walk briskly for fifteen minutes two days a week, or to test your blood glucose every other day. By starting with modest changes, you give yourself a chance to see your successes along the way and to gradually change your health habits. If you try to do too much, you may become discouraged and give up.

STEP 1: TAKING STOCK Before you can begin making changes in any area of your diabetes care, you need to know where you are in the change process for that area. The Stages of Change chart shows the main areas of diabetes management in the left-hand column. There is also a place you can add other related topics. To do a quick assessment, decide which statement along the top of the chart best describes your current "state" for each area. Place an "X" in the appropriate box.

Stages of Change

Areas of Diabetes Care	I'm thinking about it	I'm ready to start	I'm doing it	I've been doing it for six months or more
Following my food plan				
Exercising regularly				
Monitoring my blood glucose				
Taking medication as prescribed, if any				
Talking with people in my support system				
Balancing stress				
Other:_____				

STEP 2: CHOOSING CHANGE Look at your completed Stages of Change chart. Chances are you have Xs in several different columns. Notice which areas have Xs in either of the last two columns, under "I'm doing it" or "I've been doing it for six months or more." Congratulations! You are doing well in these areas of diabetes management. Continue to practice these good habits. You may also want to reread the section "Reaching and Maintaining Personal Goals" in this chapter.

Now look at the areas that have Xs in either of the first two columns, "I'm thinking about it" or "I'm ready to start." Choose which of these areas of diabetes management you would like to improve on or make progress in. For instance, if you marked "I'm ready to start" under "monitoring my blood glucose," you're ready to take action in that area.

STEP 3: PLANNING FOR ACTION In the Action Plan on page 139, write down the area you choose to make a change in. Next, fill in your long-term goal and your deadline for reaching that goal. Then, fill in a short-term goal that you can strive to achieve in the next two weeks. For example, you might decide that, two months from now, you'll be monitoring your blood glucose four times every day. For your short-term goal, you might aim to be testing twice a day by the end of two weeks, or you might set out to learn more about testing and to talk to your diabetes care team about a testing schedule. Try to foresee obstacles that might get in the way of making your change. Write these down along with ideas for avoiding or overcoming them. You may also want to review the "Taking Action" section of this chapter.

STEP 4: MONITORING YOUR PROGRESS At the end of two weeks, evaluate yourself by checking "yes" or "no" at the bottom of the Action Plan. Continue to check your progress every two weeks until you reach your long-term goal. Understand that you may have to adjust your short-term goals and expectations based on your progress or on changing circumstances in your life. Just try to keep moving in the direction of your long-term goal. Any positive change is better than no change at all. You may need several short-term goals to help you work up to accomplishing your long-term goal.

My Action Plan

The area of diabetes management I would like to improve in is:

_____

My long-term goal (___ months) is:

_____

_____

My short-term goal (two weeks) is:

_____

_____

An obstacle that may make reaching my short-term goal difficult is:

_____

To overcome this obstacle I will:

_____

_____   _____
Signature   Date

Two-week follow-up

Did I meet my short-term goal?

❏ Yes!   ❏ No

If yes, what was it that made me successful?

_____

If no, what were my obstacles? What can I do differently in the next two weeks to overcome these?

_____

_____

_____

Once you have reached your long-term goal and feel comfortable with your new habit, move on to another change. You may want to photocopy the Action Plan before you write on it so you can use it for each change you want to make.

Learning how to change your behavior to better manage your diabetes takes time. But you'll probably find that once you've improved one aspect of your diabetes care, further changes seem less difficult. This is because making lifestyle changes involves getting to know your strengths and weaknesses and learning to set reasonable goals. You can use what you've learned during one change to make future changes easier. And when you do hit rough spots, remember that you're not alone. Many people with diabetes have successfully made lifestyle changes, even those who never thought they could. Keep trying and celebrate every positive change you make—healthfully!

Key Points

- A lifestyle change is a process, not a single event. You may make progress, then relapse, then make progress again.
- You can increase your chances of success by having a plan that includes short- and long-term goals.
- If you are resisting making needed changes, you must first identify what feelings are holding you back.
- Consult books, videos, community resources, and health professionals to learn ways that others have successfully made changes.
- Recognize and avoid situations that lead to problem behaviors.
- Substitute healthy behaviors for old habits whenever possible.
- Give yourself rewards when you reach short- and long-term goals.
- Seek out support from your friends, family, and diabetes care team as you make your change.

Part Four

COMPLICATIONS AND PREVENTION

The Genetic Factor in Diabetes

If you have type II diabetes, you probably have a brother, sister, parent, grandparent, or cousin who has it, too. Certain families have a genetic background that makes them more likely to develop the insulin resistance associated with the disease. In fact, the immediate family members of a person with type II diabetes have a 40 percent chance of developing the disease.

Heredity plays a much larger role in type II diabetes than in type I. For example, if your mother has type II diabetes you have a 40 percent chance of developing type II as well. If your mother has type I diabetes, however, your risk of developing type I is no greater than four percent.

But your family members aren't necessarily destined to develop type II diabetes just because you have it. There's a lot they can do to prevent it. Following healthful habits that are similar to yours—eating balanced meals, limiting high-fat foods, exercising regularly, and managing stress— can help them reduce their risk of developing diabetes. So make your lifestyle habits a family affair!

Chapter 13

RECOGNIZING AND TREATING HEALTH PROBLEMS

You may have heard people talk about the long-term complications of diabetes. Long-term complications are those that develop gradually over a period of time. These complications can be silent and invisible, and they can become quite advanced before you even know you have them. It can take five to ten years for the complications of diabetes to cause recognizable symptoms or to be detectable in a medical examination. In fact, it is sometimes a complication of diabetes that leads to the diagnosis of type II diabetes.

The good news is that you can do a lot right now to reduce your risk of developing complications. Even if you discover some signs of complications at diagnosis or during a check-up, you can help slow down their progression.

In a recent study, researchers followed two groups of type I diabetes patients over a ten-year period.[1] One group kept their blood glucose levels as close to the normal range as possible. The other group followed a treatment plan that resulted in higher blood glucose levels. The study showed that people who had blood glucose levels closer to the normal range had a dramatic reduction in the number of complications they developed.

---

[1] Diabetes Control and Complications Trial (DCCT), National Institutes of Health, 1984-1993. In this study of 1441 patients, eye damage (retinopathy) was reduced by up to 76 percent, kidney damage (nephropathy) was reduced by up to 50 percent, and nerve damage (neuropathy) was reduced by as much as 60 percent.

Researchers think these results are important for people with type II diabetes as well because they believe many diabetes complications develop the same way in both types of diabetes. This means that you can lower your risk of complications and slow down the progress of existing complications by keeping your blood glucose levels within your target range as much as possible. That's why it's important for you to take charge of your diabetes from the very first day.

Causes of Long-term Complications

The long-term complications of diabetes are caused mainly by damage to blood vessels. The circulation of blood through the blood vessels supplies oxygen and nutrients to all parts of the body allowing the organs, tissues, and cells of the body to do their jobs. If the blood vessels become damaged, serious problems can result.

Some blood vessels are very large, others are quite small. Damage to large blood vessels (*macrovascular disease*) causes problems in the heart, brain, and feet. Damage to small blood vessels (*microvascular disease*) causes problems in the nerves, eyes, and kidneys.

Large blood vessel disease begins with some damage to or irritation of the vessel wall and then a gradual thickening of the vessel wall (called *atherosclerosis,* or hardening of the arteries). Blood fats are the main substance deposited on the vessel walls (review

TABLE 13.1 **Long-term Complications**

Complications from Large Blood Vessel Disease	Complications from Small Blood Vessel Disease
Poor circulation—gangrene or pain and cramps when walking	Nerve damage (neuropathy)—pain or loss of sensation, mainly in the feet and hands
Coronary artery disease—heart attack or angina	Eye damage (retinopathy)—blindness, cataracts, glaucoma
Carotid artery disease (arteries to brain)—stroke	Kidney damage (nephropathy)—kidney failure, high blood pressure, anemia

Chapter 2 for information about blood fats). The fat sticks to the vessel wall and builds up over time until the vessel narrows and blood flow becomes restricted. When blood flow is restricted, oxygen and nutrients cannot get to the body tissues supplied by the clogged vessels. Without oxygen and nutrients, the tissues become damaged and cannot function properly. If blood flow is completely cut off, the body tissues supplied by the blocked vessel may die. For example, if there is no blood flow to a part of the heart, then a heart attack occurs. If there is no blood flow to the toes, gangrene sets in.

How and why diabetes causes small blood vessel disease is not entirely understood, though high blood glucose levels play a major role. When glucose builds up inside the cell, it is changed to a sugar alcohol called *sorbitol*. This directly or indirectly damages the cell. Glucose may also coat proteins in the blood and in the cell tissue. This can damage the cells, causing them to stick together and become firm and inflexible. The coating also can disrupt the cells, resulting in fluid leakage or bleeding. Other factors, such as genetics, may also play some part in the development of small blood vessel problems.

Let's now look at the problems that can be caused by large and small blood vessel disease.

The Heart and Circulation

Your heart works very hard to do its job, beating an average of 100,000 times a day. Each beat of your heart sends blood carrying oxygen and nutrients through your arteries to all the parts of your body. Veins carry blood from the body back to the heart and lungs, where the blood picks up more oxygen. The heart then pumps the oxygen-rich blood back out into the body and the cycle starts all over again. The heart and the blood vessels (arteries and veins) make up your *circulatory* or *cardiovascular system*.

Large blood vessel disease can lead to heart problems, including coronary artery disease, chest pain (angina), heart attack, heart failure, or cerebrovascular disease (reduced blood flow to the brain). The later condition causes temporary strokes (called transient ischemic attacks or TIA). It could also cause a full-blown stroke, in which parts of the brain stop functioning.

Large blood vessel disease also leads to poor blood flow to the extremities, causing leg pain and cramps when walking. If the blood flow becomes very poor, the tissue dies and infection or gangrene often develops.

CORONARY ARTERY DISEASE. The blood vessels that supply the heart are called the coronary arteries. When atherosclerosis affects the coronary arteries, the flow of blood to the heart is restricted. This is called *coronary artery disease*. It can damage the heart muscle, leading to a heart attack.

Chest pain or *angina* is a warning that the blood flow to the heart may be restricted. At first angina may occur just when the heart is working harder than normal, such as during exercise. However, as the coronary arteries become more narrow, angina can occur at any time. If you have angina it does not always mean you are having a heart attack, but it is a serious sign of heart problems. Feeling unusually tired or short of breath when active, even while climbing the stairs, may also be a sign of trouble.

Your physician can check your heart health through tests and a physical examination. A common first test you may have is an electrocardiogram (EKG). This is an electrical tracing of how your heart works at rest. The EKG pattern tells if the heart muscle is in acute distress at that moment, if it is stressed or irritated, or if it has been damaged from an earlier heart attack.

If your initial screening tests are negative but there is still concern about possible heart problems, you may need a cardiac stress test. A stress test involves having an EKG and a series of blood pressure readings done while you exercise, usually on a treadmill, stationary bike, or steps. A physician can tell by the changes in the EKG during the test whether or not there is likely to be severe coronary artery disease.

An abnormal stress test or severe angina may lead your physician to suggest a cardiac catheterization, called a *coronary angiogram*. This is a test in which dye is injected into your coronary arteries to see how much blockage is present. The results will help your physician decide whether you need treatment to clear or replace damaged arteries.

Coronary artery disease is treated with medication or surgery. Medications are used to help expand the blood vessels and keep them open. If medications don't work or the vessel blockage is extreme, the blockage can be repaired through different surgical procedures. One such procedure is a *coronary bypass* operation. In this operation, the blocked vessels in the heart are replaced with blood vessels from the leg. Another procedure often used is balloon *angioplasty*, where a tube is used to insert a tiny balloon into the artery. The balloon is then inflated to expand and open the artery. A third procedure involves using lasers to direct a small, intense beam of light at the fatty deposits in the artery to clean it out and restore blood flow.

HIGH BLOOD PRESSURE AND STROKE. Almost two-thirds of adults with diabetes have high blood pressure, or *hypertension*. High blood pressure is linked to the development of coronary artery disease, heart attack, and stroke, and it can contribute to problems with the eyes and kidneys. (Eye and kidney problems are discussed later in this chapter.) High blood pressure occurs when the heart has to work hard to pump blood through narrowed blood vessels at a pressure greater than 135/85. You can read about the blood pressure test and what the numbers mean in Chapter 14.

Blood pressure can sometimes be lowered through lifestyle changes such as reducing salt and fat in the diet and increasing activity. If these don't lower the blood pressure adequately, the person will start taking medication in addition to these measures. Because high blood pressure increases the risk of diabetes complications, it needs to be treated quickly and aggressively. Therefore, blood pressure medication may be started sooner than usual for people who have diabetes. Also, it is important to find the right medication since some can actually raise blood glucose or blood fat levels. If you need blood pressure medication, talk to your physician about the side effects to make sure the medication you take is right for you.

High blood pressure is a key risk factor for stroke—another reason why it needs to be treated and controlled. Stroke is caused by blockage of the blood vessels in the brain. Because blood vessel disease and atherosclerosis are associated with diabetes, people with diabetes have a greater risk for stroke than the general population. You can lower your risk by controlling your blood pressure and cholesterol level. Lowering your blood glucose may help prevent this too, though this has not been proven yet.

POOR CIRCULATION TO THE LEGS AND FEET. When the small and large blood vessels of the legs and feet are clogged, circulation to the legs and feet is restricted. This condition, called *peripheral vascular disease,* is one of the most common problems associated with diabetes and atherosclerosis. The first signs of this problem may be discomfort or pain when standing or walking. If the blood vessel damage is not too extensive, the pain will go away after a short rest that allows circulation to be restored. In more extreme cases, peripheral vascular disease can lead to very serious leg and foot problems.

Good blood flow to the legs is especially important when you have a foot injury. Your body needs extra blood in areas where it is trying to heal or fight infection in a wound. When blood flow is poor, wounds cannot heal properly. The dangers of poor blood flow and foot injuries are increased when nerve problems are also present.

Poor circulation to the legs can be treated with medications that improve blood flow. It is also possible to have damaged blood vessels in the legs replaced with artificial blood vessels.

PREVENTION. Having diabetes does increase your risk for atherosclerosis and heart and circulation problems. That's why it is important for you to take control of your diabetes and other factors that contribute to these problems. We've discussed the need to control blood glucose and blood pressure, serious risk factors for atherosclerosis, heart attack, and stroke. Smoking, high blood fats, and being overweight can also stack up against the health of your heart and blood vessels.

People who smoke have two to four times the rate of blood vessel disease as those who do not smoke. Even if you have smoked for years, you can still lower your risk for heart disease by quitting now. If you have tried to quit without success, ask your diabetes care team to refer you to a program that may help you succeed.

For many people, heredity plays a large role in their tendency to have high blood fat (cholesterol and triglyceride) levels. Eating high-fat foods and being overweight can also contribute to high blood fat levels. The connection between heart health, blood fats, and dietary fat has been demonstrated in studies of different cultures. For example in Japan, where the typical diet is low in fat, there is a low rate of heart disease. In the United States and Finland, where people tend to eat a lot of fat, there is a high rate of heart disease. You can decrease your blood fats and your risk for heart disease by controlling your blood glucose, decreasing the fat in your diet, being active, and keeping your weight in a range that is reasonable for you. Medications may also be used.

Almost 80 percent of people with type II diabetes are overweight. If you are 20 percent or more over the weight recommended for your gender and height (see page 177), you are at greater risk for heart disease. Being overweight is also linked to high blood pressure and high blood glucose, two other risk factors for heart disease. Your treatment plan includes a food plan and exercise program that can help you lose weight if necessary. Talk to your diabetes care team about reasonable weight goals and plans to achieve them.

Reduce Your Risk of Heart and Circulation Problems

- *Don't smoke.*
- *Lower the fat and salt in your diet.*
- *Make daily activity or exercise a part of your life.*
- *Reach and remain at a reasonable weight for you.*
- *Strive to keep your blood glucose within your target range.*
- *Visit your diabetes care team two to four times a year.*

Nerves

Nerves are a communication system for your body. They work like a network of telephone lines, allowing your brain and the rest of your body to send messages back and forth. Some nerves carry messages of sensation such as pain, touch, or temperature. Others carry instructions from the brain to your legs, feet, hands, and internal organs to tell them what to do.

NEUROPATHY (NERVE DAMAGE). When your nerves are damaged, messages between your brain and other parts of your body may be distorted or may not be sent at all. High blood glucose levels over time cause neuropathy either by directly damaging nerves or by damaging the small blood vessels that supply the nerves.

There is no easy way to explain the symptoms of neuropathy. Sometimes there are no symptoms at all. Sometimes there is pain or a loss of feeling or movement in the affected area. Symptoms may develop slowly or very quickly and last anywhere from a few weeks to years. On rare occasions, symptoms seem to appear overnight and go away just as quickly.

Neuropathy happens most often in the feet and lower legs, and sometimes in the hands. Usually there is numbness, tingling, burning, and pain in the affected areas. There is sometimes a complete loss of sensation in the feet. This is an important concern because it is possible to step on a sharp object and be unaware of the injury. Coupled with poor circulation to the legs and feet, unnoticed foot injuries can quickly become infected and cause very serious problems. For this reason, daily foot inspection and care is extremely important for people with diabetes. Foot care is discussed in more detail in Chapter 14.

Internal organs including the bladder, stomach, and intestines can also be affected by neuropathy. Neuropathy in the nerves controlling the bladder can make it hard to sense whether the bladder has been emptied completely. This can lead to problems with bladder infections. Neuropathy in the nerves controlling stomach activity is called *gastroparesis.* This condition slows down the digestion of food and the emptying of the stomach, resulting in nausea, bloating, or vomiting after a meal. When the nerves to the intestines are affected, constipation or diarrhea may occur.

Carpal tunnel syndrome is another condition which affects the nerves and happens more often to people who have diabetes. This syndrome often is seen in people who use their hands to do repetitive motions, such as typing. Over time, the affected hands feel stiff and weak and hurt. Up to 30 percent of people with diabetes get carpal tunnel syndrome in one or both hands.

SEXUAL DYSFUNCTION. In normal sexual function, there are a number of mental and physical steps that prepare a man or woman for intercourse. When a man becomes excited, his brain signals the blood vessels in his penis to fill with blood. This causes his penis to become hard and erect. When a woman becomes sexually aroused, her brain signals the nerves and blood vessels in her clitoris and vagina. Her vagina becomes lubricated and ready for penetration.

Due to diabetes, some men may experience sexual dysfunction. One common problem is *retrograde ejaculation*, or an inability to ejaculate despite having an orgasm. The second and most common problem is *impotence*, or the inability to achieve or maintain an erection during sex.

These problems occur because diabetes can damage the nerves that carry signals to the blood vessels of the penis. When these nerve signals are blocked, the penis does not fill with blood or become hard. Some of the blood vessels that supply the penis may also become damaged.

Impotence related to diabetes develops slowly over many months or even years. A man may notice his erections becoming softer and less frequent. In time, he will lose his ability to become hard. Unfortunately, impotence related to diabetes cannot be reversed. Men who have diabetes can lower their risk of impotence by not smoking and by maintaining target blood glucose levels.

Sometimes men lose interest in sex as they lose their ability to have intercourse. Loss of desire may be more related to the frustration and embarrassment of impotence rather than any physical change in their sex drive.

It's important to determine the cause of impotence before deciding how to treat it. Diabetes is only one possible cause. For example, certain medicines used to treat high blood pressure cause temporary impotence. Low male hormone levels also can cause a man to lose his ability to have an erection. Finally, psychological or emotional factors may also contribute to sexual problems. A physician who specializes in treating impotence, usually a urologist, can help to identify the cause and suggest a method of treatment. A man and his partner can choose the treatment best suited to them.

There are several different medications available to treat impotence. When a medication is used, it is injected into the penis to increase blood flow and produce an erection. This may cause an erection that lasts from 30 to 90 minutes. If one of these medications is used, close follow-up with a physician is advised to assure that the medication is effective, is used correctly and safely, and that no side-effects occur.

A second treatment option is to use a vacuum device. The penis is placed in a cylinder-like sleeve. When vacuum pressure is applied, the penis fills with blood and is ready for intercourse.

A third option to treat impotence is surgical implantation of a penile prosthesis. There are two main types of implants: a semi-rigid device and an inflatable device. During surgery, a physician places one of these devices in the penis. The semi-hard device is the most popular, though it makes the penis stay semi-rigid all of the time. The inflatable device is inflated before intercourse and then it is deflated afterwards.

Sexual problems in women with diabetes have not been studied extensively, and the studies that have been done show conflicting results. Some women have reported difficulty in becoming sexually aroused or reaching orgasm. Sometimes women temporarily lose interest in sex because of health problems related to diabetes, frustration and anxiety about having diabetes, or a change in self-esteem. Talking to a health care provider or a counselor about these issues is a good first step towards coping.

For both men and women, sexual problems may require consultation with a psychologist. It may also be helpful for you and your partner to visit with a psychologist together. Though you may at first feel uncomfortable speaking with someone else about sexual problems, remember that you are not alone. Many other people with and without diabetes have experienced the same difficulties. Your diabetes care team or health care provider can refer you to a psychologist who is trained and experienced in helping people cope with sexual problems.

DETECTION, TREATMENT, AND PREVENTION OF NERVE DAMAGE. Your physician should check how your nerves are working as part of your regular diabetes care. This can be done by testing your reflexes and checking your feet and hands for decreased sensation. Your physician should ask if you have trouble emptying your bladder, problems with sexual function, or numbness, tingling or unusual pain anywhere in your body.

It can be hard to tell if pain or weakness in a part of your body is caused by neuropathy or by some other problem. If there is a question, your physician can order a test called an EMG. An EMG measures nerve impulses as they move along a nerve. For example, this test can be done on leg nerves to tell if the damage is due to diabetes or to pressure on the nerves from back problems.

The best way to treat or prevent neuropathy in any area of the body is to control your blood glucose levels. Blood glucose control may not reverse numbness or tingling, but it can slow or stop additional nerve damage. Good control can also bring on dramatic pain relief. Medications can also be used to control the symptoms of painful neuropathy and gastroparesis.

If neuropathy has caused you to lose feeling in part of your body, it is important to take extra care to avoid injury to that area. Check it daily for infections and other problems. Remember, you cannot rely on your senses to alert you to injury.

Eyes

What a marvelous creation the eyes are, yet it is easy to take them for granted. If you think about it, you depend on your eyesight for almost everything you do. It's hard to imagine living without your eyesight, but with diabetes that is a possibility you cannot afford to ignore. The blood vessels in the eyes are very sensitive to high blood glucose levels, which is one of the reasons that keeping your blood glucose within your target range is so important.

RETINOPATHY. The retina is the area of your eye where light changes into messages that are sent to your brain. Damage to the retina is called *retinopathy*. Retinopathy is potentially the most serious eye problem for people with diabetes.

Retinopathy often begins with damage to the small blood vessels of the eyes. The blood cannot flow properly and the small vessels begin to weaken and become wider in spots. The vessels begin to leak fluid, and the fluid can interfere with the retina's ability to receive images. This is called *early* or *background retinopathy* and it occurs in 80 percent of people who have had diabetes for 25 years or more. Often there are no symptoms with background retinopathy.

If early or background retinopathy is not detected and controlled, it can lead to what is called *proliferative retinopathy*. This happens because new, abnormal blood vessels develop to compensate for the clogged smaller vessels. The abnormal vessels grow on the retina or other parts of the eye. These vessels bleed easily, which may cause cloudy vision. Sometimes the blood is reabsorbed and normal vision will return; other times vision remains cloudy until this condition is treated. The bleeding may also lead to large eye hemorrhages and severe loss of vision or blindness. Even with proliferative retinopathy, you may not have symptoms until your eyes are damaged. Therefore, it is important to have an eye exam at least once a year so that retinopathy can be detected and treated as early as possible.

OTHER EYE PROBLEMS. Cataracts and glaucoma are two eye problems that affect many people as they get older. When you have diabetes, your risk for these eye problems is increased.

A cataract is a thickening or clouding of the lens of your eye. When this happens, rays of light cannot pass through to your retina. Your eyesight becomes cloudy. Cataracts can be removed in surgery and replaced with a lens that allows you to see clearly.

Glaucoma happens when you have increased pressure in your eye. The pressure can damage your retina. Eye pressure should be checked once a year as part of your yearly eye exam. If your eye pressure is too high, you can take medication to lower the pressure.

BLURRED VISION FROM HIGH BLOOD GLUCOSE. Sometimes people with diabetes have blurred vision that is not caused by proliferative retinopathy. This blurred vision is usually temporary and often happens when blood glucose levels are high, such as when you're first diagnosed with diabetes. The blurred vision is caused by high blood glucose levels or a large change in blood glucose levels.

If your blood glucose level is very high for more than a few days, changes often occur inside your eyes. First, the extra glucose causes the lenses of your eyes to swell slightly. You won't be able to tell that this is happening by looking at your eyes in a mirror. Second, the swelling prevents light rays from focusing on the retina in the usual way, thus causing blurry vision. Glasses should not be prescribed during this time because they may not be necessary or will be the wrong prescription when the vision is stabilized.

Sometimes your eyes get used to the high blood glucose levels in your body and your vision improves. However, the overall health of your eyes is still a concern. High blood glucose levels over an extended amount of time may damage your eyes permanently.

Remember, the main goal of managing your diabetes is to reach your target blood glucose level and maintain it. By doing so, you may initially experience blurry vision again because your eyes are adapting to the change. This is a temporary condition.

DETECTION, TREATMENT, AND PREVENTION. Although diabetes is one of the leading causes of blindness in adults, many people are now able to avoid this complication, thanks to new awareness, prevention, and treatment.

Everyone with diabetes should have a yearly eye exam. At the examination, your eye doctor can dilate your eyes and check your retina with any of several methods. An ophthalmoscope directs a beam of light into your eye. This allows the physician to look at the blood vessels around the retina. Your doctor may also use a microscope called a slit lamp that magnifies the inside of your eye.

If the retina looks like it is damaged, your physician may order a *fluorescein angiogram*. In this test, a dye is injected into your arm. After a few seconds it travels through the blood vessels in your eyes. Technicians take photographs of your retina as the dye flows through these vessels. The photographs show if there is leakage or abnormal blood vessels in your retina and pinpoint the exact areas that need to be treated.

Proliferative retinopathy is usually treated with laser therapy. The laser is a very small, intense beam of light. The doctor aims the laser at the leaking vessels and seals the leaks with the laser. Sometimes surgery is needed to remove blood or scar tissue from the eye or to repair damage if the retina becomes detached from its base. Laser therapy and surgery can help restore lost vision for some people. For others, it simply helps slow the progress of the retinopathy. Much will depend on when changes in the eye are discovered and treated. The sooner you discover changes and receive treatment, the better your chances of keeping your eyesight.

You can safeguard your eyesight and prevent retinopathy from progressing by keeping your blood glucose level within your target range. You can also safeguard your eyesight by keeping your blood pressure down. High blood pressure causes more leaking in damaged blood vessels.

Kidneys

Your body has two kidneys which are located in your lower abdomen near your spine. Your kidneys remove waste products from your blood and make urine. They remove the waste by filtering your blood through millions of very small blood vessels. The waste leaves your body through urination. If the small blood vessels in the kidney become damaged, kidney disease can result. One out of ten people with type II diabetes develops kidney disease.

NEPHROPATHY. Kidney disease is called *nephropathy*. It develops slowly over time, usually taking ten to fifteen years before any signs of damage are noticed. Clinical symptoms of damage do not appear until kidney disease is quite advanced.

Early kidney damage causes small amounts of a protein called *albumin* to spill into the urine. If kidney damage continues to worsen, more protein will leak into your urine. The loss of protein causes fluid to leak out of the blood vessels into the surrounding tissue. This causes a condition called *edema* in which parts of the body—usually the legs and hands—appear swollen and full. If kidney disease advances and your blood starts accumulating too many waste products (such as *urea* or *creatinine*), fatigue, loss of appetite, nausea, and vomiting may result. When the damage is too widespread, your kidneys will stop working altogether.

If both of your kidneys stop working and you are unable to clear waste products from the blood, you will need dialysis or a kidney transplant. Dialysis is a treatment in which you're hooked up to a machine that filters waste products from your blood, just as your kidneys once did. Dialysis usually takes place at a hospital or clinic. It takes about three to four hours and must be done two to three times a week. Transplanting a new kidney into a person with kidney failure due to diabetes can be very successful at reestablishing kidney function. Your age and general health will determine whether or not you're able to receive a donor kidney.

DETECTION, TREATMENT, AND PREVENTION. New tests are now available that can identify very small amounts of protein in the urine. It's a good idea to have a urine protein test, called a *microalbumin level*, at least once a year. Recent studies show that ACE inhibitors, a type of blood pressure medicine, can help treat early kidney disease. If your test for protein in the urine is positive, your physician may prescribe an ACE inhibitor or some other blood pressure medication to treat the problem.

The two best things you can do for your kidneys are to keep your blood glucose as close to your target range as possible and to control your blood pressure. Good blood glucose control can help prevent kidney disease by preventing blood vessel damage. It can also slow down kidney disease once you have it. Maintaining a healthy blood pressure is very important to preserving your kidney health as well.

Key Points

- You can reduce your risk of developing complications or slow the progression of existing complications by keeping your blood glucose levels as close to normal as possible.
- Long-term complications of diabetes are caused mainly by damage to blood vessels.
- Damage to large blood vessels can lead to coronary artery disease and other heart problems, and to poor circulation in the legs and feet.
- Smoking, being overweight, and having a family history of high blood fat levels can also contribute to heart problems.
- Damage to small blood vessels can cause nerve damage (neuropathy), eye damage (retinopathy), and kidney damage (nephropathy).
- It's important to visit your diabetes care team on a regular basis so that any complications can be recognized and treated as soon as possible.

Chapter 14

STAYING HEALTHY

As we mentioned in the introduction to this book, keeping your treatment plan running smoothly is much like keeping your car running smoothly. You are responsible for everyday maintenance of your car. You put in gas and oil, you clean the windshield, and you put air in the tires. But to keep your car in good repair, you also need to take it to a specialist on a regular basis. A specialist tunes the engine and makes sure your car is working as it should. Your diabetes treatment works in a similar way. You are responsible for your care most of the time, but you need to schedule regular visits with your diabetes care team to look at the "big picture" and to make sure your diabetes care is staying on track.

This chapter will explain the "routine maintenance" your body needs as you care for your diabetes. You'll learn what you should expect of good diabetes care and how you can prepare for your team visits. You'll become familiar with the tests and exams you should have on a regular basis. Finally, you'll learn about an aspect of your diabetes care that requires monitoring by both you and your diabetes care team—the routine care of your feet.

The Team Approach to Diabetes Care

We have spoken throughout this book of your diabetes care team. The truth is, you are the center of your diabetes care team because you follow your treatment plan and make decisions about everyday care. However, other people with special expertise are part of

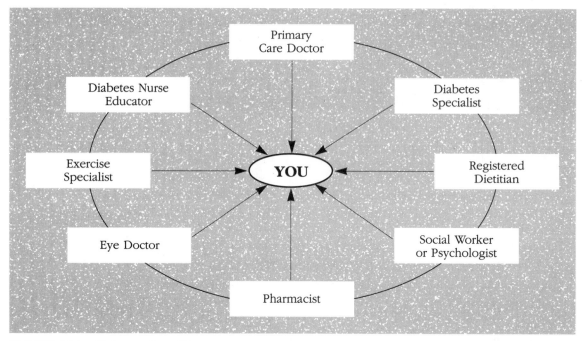

FIGURE 14.1 **Diabetes Care Team**

your team and can help you monitor and manage your care. Your diabetes care team can help you set treatment goals and timelines to reach those goals. They can outline what treatment choices you have, teach you self-care skills, help you solve problems, and evaluate how your diabetes treatment is working.

Your diabetes care team may include some or all of the following health professionals:

Primary Care Doctor. This doctor is trained to take care of all common health problems. He or she will lead your diabetes care team and help you make decisions about your treatment.

Diabetes Specialist. This is a doctor who specializes in treating diabetes. Diabetes specialists are often doctors with special training in the body's endocrine system (endocrinologists). You and your primary care doctor may consult with a diabetes specialist when special knowledge is needed in your treatment.

Diabetes Nurse Educator. This person's job is to teach you all about diabetes and how to take care of yourself. Topics include blood glucose monitoring, recognizing and treating low blood glucose levels, and managing your diabetes during an illness. If you need to take insulin, your diabetes nurse educator may help your physician decide what dose you need and will teach you how to take it. A diabetes nurse educator is usually certified by the American Association of Diabetes Educators as a certified diabetes educator (CDE).

Registered Dietitian. This team member helps you design a food plan that is right for your lifestyle and that suits your tastes. Your dietitian will also help you make changes in your eating, shopping, and cooking habits if needed. Often, dietitians who work in the diabetes field are also certified diabetes educators.

Exercise Specialist. This person helps you identify physical activities you enjoy and assists you in designing a safe and effective exercise program.

Social Worker or Psychologist. This team member helps you and your family work through any problems you may have adjusting to or living day-to-day with your diabetes. He or she helps you deal with personal, family, and work issues that affect your health or your ability to take care of yourself.

Pharmacist. Pharmacists can help you learn about diabetes medications and the other supplies you need to take care of your diabetes. Your pharmacist can also help you understand how various drugs interact and how they might affect you.

Other specialists help monitor for complications:

- An *eye doctor* (ophthalmologist) will give you eye exams and monitor any changes in your eyes.
- A *podiatrist* will help take care of your feet, including cutting your toenails if you're unable to do so, or treating corns and calluses if they develop.
- A *nephrologist* will help with kidney problems if they occur.
- A *urologist* will help with sexual function problems if they occur.

WHAT TO EXPECT FROM YOUR TEAM. At each visit, a member of your team will ask if you are having any problems following any part of your treatment plan, any symptoms of low or high blood glucose levels, or any symptoms of complications. Your blood glucose monitoring records will also be reviewed and discussed, and routine blood tests will be done that will help you and your team know if your treatment is working. Your team will also check your weight, blood pressure, and feet, paying particular attention to nerve responses and pulses. If you have goals for your blood pressure and your cholesterol and triglyceride levels, you and your team will discuss these as well.

You and your team can evaluate whether you are meeting your treatment goals. If your goals are being met, you will probably continue with your current treatment plan. If your goals are not being met, your treatment plan may need to be changed or the goals reassessed. If necessary you will be referred to one of the specialists on the team for the care you need.

HOW OFTEN TO SEE YOUR TEAM. When you are diagnosed with diabetes, you need to visit your diabetes care team as often as necessary to learn about food planning, blood glucose monitoring, and exercise, and to get your blood glucose levels into your target range. At first, you may talk to certain members of your team as often as every one to two weeks to make needed adjustments.

After the initial adjustment period, you need to schedule diabetes care visits with your care team two to four times per year. Visits may be scheduled more often if your blood glucose or blood pressure goals are not being met, if you are having any signs of complications, or if you have other immediate problems.

The Physical Tune-Up

As part of your visits with your diabetes care team, you will take a series of tests that help you monitor your diabetes treatment and your health. The Physical Tune-Up on pages 164–165 shows a year-long schedule for all the tests and exams needed for good diabetes care. Each of the tests is explained in more detail later in this section. Use the Tune-Up to record your test results and to remind yourself when it's time for a diabetes care visit. The blank spaces show when you should have each test. Write your results in these spaces. You do not need to fill in the shaded areas.

The recommended times for each test are based on American Diabetes Association standards and reflect the minimum care you should expect from your diabetes care team. Your health care provider may ask you to come in more often or to have some tests done more often, depending on your individual needs. If you notice that you are not being given a test you need as often as the Tune-Up recommends, call this to the attention of your team.

HEMOGLOBIN A$_{1c}$ (HbA$_{1c}$). This test tells you your average blood glucose level over the past six to ten weeks. The HbA$_{1c}$ test is important because the results, along with your blood glucose records, help you and your diabetes care team know whether your treatment plan is working. There is no universal "normal" HbA$_{1c}$ result, because the methods for measuring HbA$_{1c}$ differ from laboratory to laboratory. Check what the normal range is for your lab. Then decide with your diabetes care team what your target HbA$_{1c}$ is. Be sure to have this test done every three to six months. Without the results from this test, it's hard to know if your treatment is on the right track.

BLOOD PRESSURE. Blood pressure is the force pushing blood through your body. When blood pushes very hard against the walls of the arteries, you can develop high blood pressure (hypertension). This puts extra strain on your heart and can lead to heart disease. Blood pressure is recorded as two numbers. The first (upper) number is the *systolic pressure*; this is the pressure in your blood vessels when the heart contracts. The second (lower) number is the *diastolic pressure*; this is the pressure in your vessels when the heart is relaxed.

TOTAL CHOLESTEROL. Cholesterol is a waxy substance found in food and made in the body. Your body needs cholesterol for some body functions, but too much total cholesterol can increase your risk of heart disease. Total cholesterol measures all the cholesterol in your blood. This includes HDL-cholesterol and LDL-cholesterol.

HDL-CHOLESTEROL. This is a measure of the HDL-cholesterol (high density lipoprotein cholesterol) in your blood. HDL-cholesterol is often called "good" cholesterol because it carries cholesterol out of the arteries. This helps protect you against heart disease. It's good to have a high percentage of HDL-cholesterol in your blood. Regular exercise, weight loss, and blood glucose control can often increase HDL levels.

Physical Tune-Up

Check Points	Target	Yearly Checkup Date:	
Height _____ Weight _____			
Blood Pressure	Under 130/85		
HbA$_{1c}$	Within 1.5% of upper limit of lab normal		
Total Cholesterol	Under 200 mg/dl		
HDL-Cholesterol	35 mg/dl or more (men) 45 mg/dl or more (women)		
Cholesterol/HDL Ratio	4.5 or under		
LDL-Cholesterol	Under 130 mg/dl		
Triglycerides	Under 200 mg/dl		
Urine Protein	See table on page 166		
EKG (electrocardiogram)	Normal		
Thyroid Function	T4 4.5 – 12.5 µg/dL TSH 0.2 – 5.50 µIU/mL		
Dental Exam			
Foot Exam			
Eye Exam			
Meter Check			
Observe Injection (if taking insulin)			

Target ranges for elderly may vary, so check with your health care provider.

Physical Tune-Up from *Owner's Manual Type II,* Staged Diabetes Management, © 1995 International Diabetes Center, Institute for Research and Education HealthSystem Minnesota

	Visits with your health care provider should be at least two to four times a year.		
3 Month Visit Date:	**6 Month Visit** Date:	**9 Month Visit** Date:	**Yearly Checkup** Date:

CHOLESTEROL/HDL RATIO. This test can help determine your risk of heart disease. Your cholesterol/HDL ratio tells how much of your total cholesterol is HDL-cholesterol, or "good" cholesterol. Even if your total cholesterol is normal but your HDL level is low, you're still at risk for heart disease. To find your ratio, divide your total cholesterol by your HDL-cholesterol. A low ratio means you have lower risk of heart disease. A high ratio means you have a higher risk of heart disease.

LDL-CHOLESTEROL. This is a measure of the LDL-cholesterol (low density lipoprotein cholesterol) in your blood. LDL carries cholesterol in the bloodstream. It's often called "bad" cholesterol because it can stick to the walls of your blood vessels. This makes the opening in the vessels smaller so it's hard for the blood to flow through. Smaller blood vessel openings can lead to heart problems. It's good to have *less* of this kind of cholesterol in your body.

TRIGLYCERIDES. This is a measure of the triglycerides (fats) in your blood. Triglycerides are fats that are both found in food and made by the body. High triglyceride levels put you at greater risk for heart disease. Triglyceride levels can go up when blood glucose levels are high. High-fat, high-sugar foods and alcohol can also increase triglyceride levels.

URINE PROTEIN. Urine protein is a way to monitor kidney function. The table shows all the different tests that measure protein in your urine. If your urine has protein in it, your health care provider may want to do other tests to check your kidney function.

Urine Protein Tests Available	Normal
Random Albumin (µg/mL)	less than 20
Albumin/Creatinine Ratio (mg/gm)	less than 30
Timed Microalbumin Excretion Rate (µg/min)	less than 20
24-hour Microalbumin Excretion (mg/24 hour)	less than 30
24-hour Total Protein (mg/day)	less than 165

EKG (ELECTROCARDIOGRAM). This is a test to check how your heart is functioning and to see if there are any problems.

Sometimes this test is done while you walk on a treadmill, which is called a stress EKG, exercise EKG, or stress test.

THYROID FUNCTION. This is a blood test that shows your levels of thyroid hormone (T4) and thyroid stimulating hormone (TSH). T4 regulates how your body uses energy. TSH regulates the release of T4 by your thyroid gland. If your T4 is below normal and your TSH is above normal, there is not enough thyroid hormone in your blood. This is called hypothyroidism. If your T4 is above normal and your TSH is below normal, you have too much thyroid hormone in your blood. This is called hyperthyroidism. Diabetes increases your risk of developing hypothyroidism or hyperthyroidism.

EYE EXAM. An eye exam is done by an ophthalmologist. Your eyes will be dilated (opened) with a medication so that the retina, or the back of the eye, can easily be seen. This is where eye changes from diabetes can occur. The ophthalmologist tests your vision and also tests your eyes for glaucoma.

FOOT EXAM. This is done by your health care provider or by a podiatrist. Your feet are checked for any sores, cracks, infection, or other changes. The blood vessels and nerves in your feet are checked, too.

DENTAL EXAM. This exam is done by a dentist and a dental hygienist. A dental exam includes cleaning your teeth and examining them for decay and checking your gums for signs of gum disease.

BLOOD GLUCOSE AND METER CHECK. Once a year, compare a test you do on your meter against a laboratory blood glucose test. The comparison will tell you if you are getting accurate results from your testing method. See page 81 for more information on how to do this comparison.

Preparing for Your Visits

To get the most from your visits with your diabetes care team, you need to be prepared—you need to know as much as possible about your own health *before* you go. Keep a list of your questions and concerns between visits. If there is something about your health that is bothering you, your check-up is the time to talk about it. Think about the different areas of care, and be ready to discuss them with your diabetes care team.

The form on page 169 includes questions to help you prepare for your visits. Your answers to these questions will give your team members important information that can help them help you. Copy the form and fill it out before each visit. There is also a space for you to write down questions that you want to ask your team members.

Caring for Your Feet

Another aspect of diabetes care that requires regular attention from both you and your team is caring for your feet. People with diabetes are at high risk for foot problems.

Foot problems begin because of lack of feeling and decreased blood flow in the legs. A lack of feeling can cause you not to notice a callous, blister, or other injury. Left unattended, the sore spot can become infected. If blood flow is restricted because of blood vessel damage, your ability to fight off infections decreases. Without plenty of oxygen and nutrients provided by blood, a sore or injury cannot heal. Also, bacteria thrive on glucose and are more likely to cause infection in people with high blood glucose levels.

A skin infection that is left untreated can quickly turn to a condition called *gangrene,* in which areas of body tissue die. Gangrene cannot be reversed. The only treatment is to cut away the dead tissue by amputation. Each year there are more than 55,000 amputations among Americans who have diabetes. Experts believe that more than half of these amputations can be avoided with proper foot care.

You can decrease your risk of developing hard-to-heal foot infections by keeping your blood glucose levels within your target range and by caring for your feet every day. Call your diabetes care team whenever you have a foot injury, callous, or blister that doesn't heal in a reasonable amount of time.

PROPER FOOT CARE. Wash your feet every day with warm water and mild soap and dry them with a soft towel, making sure to dry between your toes. Check your feet every day to look for cracks,

My Diabetes Care Visits

Food Plan Am I having trouble with any part of my food plan? Does it fit my lifestyle? Am I gaining or losing weight? Are there certain foods I have questions about?_____
_____
_____

Exercise What do I do for exercise? How often do I exercise? How long? What times of the day? How has exercise made a difference in my blood glucose readings?_____
_____
_____

Medications What is my current regimen? Has there been a change since my last visit? Am I taking my medications as prescribed?_____
_____

Blood Tests How often am I testing my blood glucose? What times of the day? Are the results in my target range?_____
_____

Hyperglycemia (high blood glucose) Am I urinating more than usual? Do I have to get up from sleep several times to go to the bathroom? Am I always thirsty?_____
_____

Hypoglycemia (low blood glucose) How often and when does my blood glucose get low? How do I feel? What do I do to feel better? Do I usually carry a carbohydrate food with me?_____
_____
_____

Illness Have I been sick since my last visit? What was wrong? How was the illness treated? Do I have questions about what to watch for when I'm sick? Do I know who to call with any concerns?
_____
_____

Unusual Stress What is happening in my life? How do I feel? Has this affected my blood glucose levels?_____
_____

Complications Am I having problems seeing? Do I have burning or numbness in my hands or feet? Am I having sexual problems?_____
_____

My Questions_____
_____
_____
_____

blisters, infections, and injuries. You often can see a problem before you can feel it, and this is expecially true if you've experienced any loss of feeling. Use a mirror or magnifying glass if you are unable to look at the bottoms of your feet easily. If you cannot check your own feet, have someone do it for you.

If you do notice a minor break in the skin on your feet, treat it right away. Wash the area with soap and water, then dry and cover it with clean gauze or a bandage. Watch for signs of infection such as redness, swelling, warmth, pain, or oozing. If you notice any of these signs, or if the break doesn't heal within a reasonable amount of time, call your diabetes care team.

Moisturize dry skin on your feet with a cream or lotion. If the cream or lotion causes redness or other problems, stop using it and tell your health care provider. Clip your toenails straight across. Be careful not to trim them too short or to allow them to grow too long. Use a cardboard emory board to smooth down sharp toenail edges.

Proper foot care also means choosing the right footware. Many people wear uncomfortable shoes in the name of style and suffer only minor discomfort as a result. But for people with diabetes,

Foot Care No-Nos

DO NOT soak your feet. Soaking dries skin and creates cracks. Cracks allow germs to enter and could lead to infection. Soaking also slows down healing.

DO NOT use hot water bottles or heating pads or any electrical device to heat or massage your feet.

DO NOT smoke. Smoking reduces blood flow to your feet.

DO NOT sit with your legs crossed. Anything that slows blood flow to your feet can be harmful.

DO NOT wear knee-high stockings that are too tight.

DO NOT perform "bathroom surgery" by using razor blades, scissors, or sandpaper on your feet.

DO NOT use over-the-counter wart or corn removers on your feet. Talk to your diabetes care team if you want a growth removed.

DO NOT go barefoot, even indoors.

shoes that don't fit well can restrict blood flow to the feet, which can be dangerous. Choose shoes with a fit that is snug but not tight. Shoes should have a soft insole and inner lining, free of rough areas and thick seams. The toe should be wide and shaped like your foot; it should not pinch. The end of the shoe should be one-half inch longer than your longest toe when you are standing. Shoes made of leather or cotton are better than those made of synthetic materials because they allow your foot to "breathe." Always wear shoes or slippers, even around the house.

As with other aspects of your health care, your diabetes care team can help you in caring for your feet. Ask your team to check your feet during your regular visits. At some point you may need to see a podiatrist for help with ingrown toenails, corns, callouses, trimming thick toenails, or if you need special shoes.

Whenever you experience problems with foot care or with any other aspect of your diabetes, be assertive in seeking out help. Your diabetes care team is there to act as a resource and a support system for you, whether your treatment is running smoothly or not. Like many people with diabetes, you may be tempted to avoid visits with your team if your blood glucose levels are high or if you are having trouble following your treatment plan. You may fear that you will "fail" your tests and exams. But your team is there to help you, not to grade your results and pass judgment on you.

As the key member of your team, you are responsible for monitoring your diabetes care. This includes monitoring the health professionals you work with to be sure you are receiving the care you need from them. And they can help you best when you are an active, informed team member yourself.

Key Points

- Visit with your diabetes care team at least two to four times a year so they can check on your health, answer any questions you have, and help you adjust your treatment plan if needed.
- To get the most from your visits with your team, think about how your treatment is going and write down any questions or concerns before you go.
- To care for your feet and avoid complications, check your feet daily for injuries or other problems, wear well-fitting shoes, and have your health care provider check your feet at each visit.
- Use the Physical Tune-Up to monitor your diabetes care and your health.

Chapter 15

RESEARCH AND PREVENTION

Today, people with diabetes can expect to live long and healthy lives. Beginning with the discovery of insulin in 1921, scientists and researchers have advanced the knowledge of diabetes to an astounding level. We now know more than ever before about how diabetes develops and what altered chemical and body processes characterize diabetes. This knowledge translates into more discoveries, and these discoveries lead to continued improvements in the prevention, management, and outcome of diabetes.

Preventing Diabetes in Your Family

People with diabetes often worry that their children or siblings will develop diabetes. Type II diabetes *does* tend to run in families, and the risk of developing it is especially significant if an immediate family member—parent, brother, or sister—has diabetes.

Relative with Type II Diabetes	Family Member's Risk
Brother or Sister	40%
Mother or Father	40%
Both Mother and Father	70%

A person is also more likely to develop diabetes if he or she:

- is African American/Black, American Indian, Alaskan Native, Hispanic, Pacific Islander, or Asian;
- is overweight;
- is over 40 years of age;
- has abnormal blood fats;
- has high blood pressure;
- has a history of diabetes during pregnancy (gestational diabetes);
- has given birth to a baby weighing over nine pounds; or
- has a sedentary lifestyle.

But having one, or even many, of these risk factors does not necessarily mean a family member will develop diabetes. Researchers believe that diabetes can be prevented or delayed by making a series of lifestyle changes aimed at reducing risk factors. Of course, your family members can't change their family history or genetic makeup, but they can make changes that will have a positive effect in other areas of health risk. Any improvement can make a difference.

By now you may have guessed that the lifestyle changes that help reduce the risk of diabetes are the very things we've been discussing throughout this whole book—eating healthfully, being active, balancing stress, and managing weight. That's why we say that your entire family can benefit by following your example as you care for your diabetes. The advice you receive as part of your diabetes care is good advice for anyone wanting to live a long and healthy life.

It is important for family members of people with diabetes to understand their risk and to actively monitor their health. In addition to making the lifestyle changes mentioned earlier, people at risk need to let their doctors know what their risk factors are and ask for help with prevention efforts. Regular blood glucose screenings are an essential part of medical care for people at risk. Also, doctors should be asked to pay special attention to blood fats, blood pressure, and even slight elevations of blood glucose.

There are no guarantees that diabetes will be prevented by taking the measures discussed here. However, studies show that even a moderate, maintained weight loss and a minimum of regular exercise can result in decreased or delayed onset of diabetes in people who are at risk. You can encourage your family members by setting a good example—practice the healthful habits that help to treat AND prevent diabetes. It may be the best thing you can do for those you love.

A short risk assessment appears on the following page. Ask your family members to take it and to take charge of their health.

Improving Diabetes Treatment

Diabetes research is a dynamic field occupying some of the finest medical minds in the world. Current areas of research include new insulins and glucose-lowering pills that will better control blood glucose levels, other medications that will help reduce the severity of diabetes complications, new methods of monitoring diabetes care, and the genetics of diabetes. You will see and benefit from the results of this research in the years to come, even as new research is begun and the cycle continues.

NEW MEDICATIONS. Since weight is so closely linked to type II diabetes, much research has focused on ways to facilitate weight loss. Achieving and maintaining a reasonable weight is a primary goal in the treatment of type II diabetes because weight loss helps improve blood glucose levels, yet losing weight is very difficult for many people (not just people with diabetes). To address this problem, researchers are currently developing a drug that blocks the absorption of fat from the intestine. When the fat is not absorbed, the body cannot use the calories supplied by the fat. This results in weight loss and, ultimately, improved blood glucose control. Research continues on the long-term safety of other weight-loss drugs that could eventually help people with diabetes.

Aldose reductase inhibitors are another area of drug research. These drugs block the harmful effects of glucose on blood vessels. They work by blocking the action of an enzyme that converts glucose into another sugar called sorbitol. Some studies have linked sorbitol made in the body to increased blood vessel damage in the eyes, kidneys, and nerves—common complications seen in diabetes. It is believed that aldose reductase inhibitors will help prevent or minimize this damage. Researchers are also studying a

Are You at Risk?

Take the first step now to help prevent diabetes from entering your life. Answer the following questions to determine your greatest areas of risk. The more "yes" answers, the greater your risk. Any "yes" answer means you should take preventive measures now. Following the advice given in this book about eating healthfully and staying active may help delay or prevent the onset of diabetes.

Forty percent of the children or siblings of people diagnosed with type II diabetes will eventually develop diabetes unless they take steps to prevent it. Does your parent, brother, or sister have diabetes?
❑ Yes ❑ No

People in some ethnic groups have two to three times the risk of developing diabetes compared to all people. Are you African American/Black, American Indian, Alaskan Native, Hispanic, or Asian/Pacific Islander?
❑ Yes ❑ No

More than 40 percent of people with diabetes have abnormal blood fat levels. This increases their risk of heart disease up to four times that of the general population. Do you have abnormal cholesterol or blood fat?
❑ Yes ❑ No ❑ Don't Know

The longer you are overweight and the more overweight you are, the greater your risk for diabetes. Is your weight more than or equal to the weight listed in the chart for your height? (The chart on page 177 shows weights that are 20 percent over ideal weights.)
❑ Yes ❑ No

Sixty percent of people with undiagnosed diabetes have high blood pressure. Do you have high blood pressure or take blood pressure medication?
❑ Yes ❑ No ❑ Don't Know

Thirty-five to 60 percent of women who develop diabetes during pregnancy, or who have a baby over nine pounds, go on to develop type II diabetes. Did you have high blood glucose (sugar) during a pregnancy, or have a baby over nine pounds?
❑ Yes ❑ No

People who exercise three to five times a week can reduce their risk of diabetes up to 40 percent. Do you exercise (walk, garden, bike) *less than* three times a week?
❑ Yes ❑ No

drug called aminoguanidine, which may help prevent complications by blocking harmful effects of excess sugar build up in the body's tissues.

MONITORING. This is a crucial area of diabetes care and diabetes research. If you don't monitor your blood glucose levels and record the results, you and your diabetes care team cannot make judgments about your care. Yet diabetes professionals know that it is difficult to maintain a habit of regular monitoring and record-keeping. Researchers know it too and are working hard on ways to make it easier, such as the oft-promised "no-stick" blood testing device. The device furthest along uses a beam of infrared light to detect and measure glucose in blood

Weight Chart
(shows 20% over maximum ideal weights without shoes or clothing)

Women		Men	
Height	Weight	Height	Weight
4'9"	127 lbs.	5'2"	151 lbs.
4'10"	131 lbs.	5'3"	155 lbs.
4'11"	134 lbs.	5'4"	158 lbs.
5'0"	138 lbs.	5'5"	163 lbs.
5'1"	142 lbs.	5'6"	168 lbs.
5'2"	146 lbs.	5'7"	174 lbs.
5'3"	151 lbs.	5'8"	179 lbs.
5'4"	157 lbs.	5'9"	184 lbs.
5'5"	162 lbs.	5'10"	190 lbs.
5'6"	167 lbs.	5'11"	196 lbs.
5'7"	172 lbs.	6'0"	202 lbs.
5'8"	176 lbs.	6'1"	208 lbs.
5'9"	181 lbs.	6'2"	214 lbs.
5'10"	186 lbs.	6'3"	220 lbs.

vessels under the skin. In addition, great strides have been made recently in the use of computers to analyze blood glucose data. Many computer programs are already available for use in health care clinics and with personal computers. Along with meters that store data, these tools provide seamless, accurate blood glucose data collection and analysis. There are also computer programs that analyze food and activity records. See page 180 for examples of these programs and a listing of other computer resources. Also, ask your diabetes care team or look on the shelves at your local computer store for new products that can help you.

A Final Word

Caring for your diabetes requires tremendous knowledge and involvement on your part. It can often seem that other people, including your diabetes care team, just don't understand what you face. Piles of information are heaped on you and then you are seemingly left to your own devices to try to make sense of it and put it into practice in your life.

Remember, you are not alone. We urge you to *get involved*. Find reliable sources of information and appropriate health care. Seek the help and support of your team members, family, and friends as you continue to practice and refine your self care. *Stay informed* and use the resources available to you. Our knowledge about diabetes is constantly changing, and your diabetes care needs will change over time based on your health goals, your lifestyle, and other factors. Besides your diabetes care team, there are diabetes education programs, support groups, and organizations that can help you stay in touch and stay on top of your care. (See page 179 for a listing of some of these groups.) Lastly, *become a resource* to others by becoming involved in community diabetes activities and support groups.

Finally, we hope that this book will be a source of inspiration and support in your efforts to live *well* with diabetes.

RESOURCES

Diabetes Associations/Centers

International Diabetes Center Affiliates, 3800 Park Nicollet Boulevard, Minneapolis, MN 55416, (612) 993-3393

American Diabetes Association, 1660 Duke Street, Alexandria, VA 22314, (800) 232-3472

Canadian Diabetes Association, 15 Ontario Street, Suite 800, Toronto, ON M5C2E3 Canada, (416) 363-3373

National Diabetes Information Clearinghouse, 1 Information Way, Bethesda, MD 20892

Resources to Help You Find Health Care

American Association of Diabetes Educators, 444 North Michigan Avenue, Suite 1240, Chicago, IL 60611, (312) 644-2233 or (800) 338-3633

The American Dietetic Association, 216 West Jackson Boulevard, Suite 800, Chicago, IL 60606, (312) 899-0040 or (800) 877-1600

American Board of Podiatric Surgery, 1601 Dolores Street, San Francisco, CA 94110, (415) 826-3200

Impotence Institute of America, 10400 Little Patuxent Parkway, Suite 485, Columbia, MD 21044, (800) 669-1603

National Association of Social Workers, 750 First Street NE, Suite 700, Washington, DC 20002, (202) 408-8600 or (800) 638-8799

National Eye Care Project, (800) 222-3937

For the Visually Impaired

American Council of the Blind, 1155 15th Street NW, Suite 720, Washington, DC 20005, (202) 467-5081 or (800) 424-8666

Division for the Blind and Visually Impaired, Rehabilitation Service Administration, Department of Education, Mary Switzer Building, Room 3229, 330 C Street SW, Washington, DC 20202, (202) 205-9316

National Federation of the Blind, 1800 Johnson Street, Baltimore, MD 21230, (410) 659-9314

Medical Identification Aids

Medic Alert, (800) 432-5378

Life Alert, (403) 258-0822

Iden-Tag, (410) 602-1911

Emergency Medical Identification, (608) 328-8381

For Travelers

International Association for Medical Assistance to Travelers, 350 5th Avenue, Suite 5620, New York, NY 10001, (716) 754-4883

International Diabetes Federation, 40 Washington Street, B-1050 Brussels, Belgium

Computer Resources

Blood Glucose Analysis Software

These programs allow you to download or hand enter and analyze your blood glucose. Call the software manufacturer to see if the software will work with your meter.

One Touch Utility Software, Lifescan, Inc., Milpitas, CA 95035, (800) 227-8862

Mellitus Manager, Eumedix, Inc., P.O. Box 720278, San Diego, CA 92172, (800) 455-4105

BioStore, BioStore Technologies, P.O. Box 800766, Santa Clarita, CA 91380, (805) 288-1301

Glucostats Plus, Computer Specialties, Box 1581, Fairfield, CT 06430, (203) 371-5171

The Internet

http://www.diabetesnet.com General information on diabetes
http://www.niddk.nih.gov/ National Institutes of Health
http://www.adatx.org/ American Diabetes Association

INDEX